THE STRESS RX

TRUPTI GOKANI, MD

THE STRESS RX

A Neurologist's Ayurvedic Prescription for Happiness and Health

Library of Congress Control Number: 2025902811
ISBN: 978-1-964686-36-3 (paperback) 978-1-964686-37-0 (ebook)

Although this publication is designed to provide accurate information about the subject matter, the publisher and the author assume no responsibility for any errors, inaccuracies, omissions, or inconsistencies herein. This publication is intended as a resource; however, it is not intended as a replacement for direct and personalized professional services.

This book does not provide medical, psychiatric, or psychological diagnosis, treatment, or advice. It is for informational purposes only. The dietary and nutritional recommendations described in this book are not intended to substitute for medical advice. Never disregard medical, psychiatric, or psychological advice or treatment and never delay in seeking it because of anything you read in this book. Any questions that you may have regarding the diagnosis or treatment of a medical condition or any product or supplement described in this book should be directed to a qualified healthcare professional.

All matters concerning your health require ongoing medical supervision. If you have a known or suspected medical, psychiatric, or psychological condition, or are taking medications or supplements of any kind, you should consult a qualified healthcare professional before following any of the suggestions described in this book. Any dosages described in this book are intended only as guidelines. You need to consult with your healthcare professional before you use any suggestions found in this book.

The author and publisher do not warrant that this book or any information contained in it can be relied upon for applicability to any purpose or treatment, including those described in this book as typical applications for any given supplement or product. With respect to any supplements or products described in this book, the author disclaims any and all warranties, either expressed or implied, including fitness for a particular purpose.

Editors: Deborah Froese, Devon Lord
Cover and Interior Design: Emma Elzinga

Printed in the United States of America

First Edition

3 West Garden Street, Ste. 718
Pensacola, FL 32502
www.indigoriverpublishing.com

Ordering Information:

Quantity sales: Special discounts are available on quantity purchases by corporations, associations, and others. For details, contact the publisher at the address above.

Orders by US trade bookstores and wholesalers: Please contact the publisher at the address above.

With Indigo River Publishing, you can always expect great books, strong voices, and meaningful messages. Most importantly, you'll always find . . . *words worth reading.*

Table of Contents

Acknowledgements

First and foremost, I would like to express my deepest gratitude to my dear husband, Binal, whose unwavering support, patience, and encouragement carried me through the long journey of writing this book. What began during the pandemic stretched far beyond our expectations, and I could not have done it without his steady presence.

To my wonderful children, Ariya and Arman, thank you for allowing me to share pieces of your journeys within these pages. Your encouragement and unwavering belief in my voice have given me the confidence to express myself fully and without hesitation.

This book would not have been possible without the many incredible patients, coaching clients, family, friends, and colleagues who have inspired me along the way. Your stories, resilience, and trust have fueled my passion for writing and sharing these learnings.

I am also deeply grateful to Indigo Publishing for their dedication and meticulous attention to detail, ensuring that this manuscript reached the world only when it was truly ready. Their commitment to excellence has been invaluable in bringing this book to life.

Finally, I offer my heartfelt thanks to the divine, whose guidance, reassurance, and signs have continually reminded me that I am on the right path. For all the moments of clarity, inspiration, and unseen support, I am profoundly grateful.

With love and gratitude,
Trupti

Introduction

You likely turned to this book because you are struggling to embrace life fully. Your struggle may appear as overwhelm, anxiety, pain, digestive issues, or hormone imbalances, just to name a few possibilities. Stress is likely at the bottom of it.

I know because I've been there.

Stress is a tricky word. It's thrown around so easily that it has become part of the everyday vernacular, one of those catchphrases used to embody a hard-to-define sense of unease. On the one hand, some people don't identify themselves as stressed simply because they don't know what it feels like to NOT be stressed (that was me). Many live in a constant state of imbalance, unaware of the pressure they're under. On the other hand, some people believe their lives are under constant stress. When asked how they are doing, the automatic response is, "I am stressed," or "My life is so stressful."

No matter who you are, your life is impacted by stress—but it isn't all bad. Short-term stress can be good; the chemical reaction it triggers in your body increases alertness, improves performance, and activates memory receptors. That works really well when certain situations requiring your full attention arise, such as a work deadline or a medical emergency.

Long-term stress is another story, however. The continual onslaught of stress-related chemicals can lead to mental exhaustion, physical deterioration, illness, or, as with me, insomnia.

Stress—the long-term kind—knocked on my door when I was a first-year medical student, appearing to me as insomnia. (At some level, this was not so bad, as it led me to study Ayurveda!) I didn't recognize stress as the causal factor until I began digging deeper and taking a good, hard look at how the pressures in my life affected my body, mind, and spirit. Becoming a patient while training to become a doctor was a powerful experience. Since I had not been fully trained in the Western model, I was still open to other ways of approaching health and disease.

Dissatisfied by what the American health care system had to offer, I began a quest. Since this was the pre-internet era, resources were limited, so I turned to the local bookstore and read books by Andrew Weil, Deepak Chopra, and Bernie Siegel. Despite the fact that all three were trained in Western medicine, each of these brilliant physicians had the courage to step beyond mainstream, conventional thinking. They found integrative health solutions for the whole person, not just the physical body.

The Western model of medicine, as it is taught in medical school, excludes many pieces of the health care puzzle. This is a fact. Because of misguided approaches and policies, we are now experiencing a worsening state of crisis. I am truly frightened about where modern medicine is headed if we continue in this direction.

In 2020, the United States spent $4.1 trillion on health care,[1] up from $3.6 trillion in 2018.[2] While the COVID-19 pandemic certainly played a role in this, an aging population is also putting pressure on the health care system.[3] Health care costs are projected to reach $7.2 trillion annually by 2031.[4] If higher spending meant better outcomes, I might be okay with it, but this has not been the case. We are sicker than ever as a nation. In the last couple years alone, our life expectancy has fallen by more than two years.[5]

Something needs to change—and change fast, before it is too late.

Over the years, we seem to have forgotten the benefit (and cost-effectiveness) of preventative medicine and holistic care. Most people wait until symptoms are severe before they consider making an appointment with their doctors. I once asked a patient why she waited so long to see a neurologist for a tremor in her hand. It turned out that because her symptoms were infrequent and mild, she was afraid she might insult her doctor by "wasting" his time.

This, to me, is the essence of why America has become the number one health care spender in the world—with some of the worst outcomes. Patients postpone visiting the doctor for fear of receiving a disturbing diagnosis or having to pay for an expensive prescription. Doctors are trained to diagnose problems and address the symptoms with medication or surgery. Most do not pursue causation or offer preventative measures.

If symptoms are mild, they believe they should wait.

Is that you?

I sought answers and found them in Ayurveda, the ancient holistic science of self-healing. I want to share with you what I've learned, what I have witnessed by caring for my patients. That's what this book is all about.

The Stress Rx is composed of fourteen chapters. The first dives into what true health really means. The others illuminate one novel holistic concept at a time to allow a deeper understanding of yourself and why you currently struggle. Each chapter ends with action steps that include self-care exercises or self-assessment quizzes and provides directions for balancing the concept in question.

In these pages, you'll learn to recognize how and where you carry stress in your mind and body, with a specific emphasis on the gut-brain connection. Using a blend of ancient wisdom and concepts from neurolinguistic programming, you'll find the tools you need to create a balanced mind, body, and spiritual state.

I'm also sharing two formulas I utilize in my private practice and in group settings:

1. The three brain model explores the *thinking* brain (CNS or central nervous system), the *feeling* brain (ENS or enteric nervous system) and the *doing* brain (microbiome). It demonstrates how to achieve higher levels of health in mind, body, and spirit so you can live in the happiness and bliss you are meant for.

2. The SOUL Method shares a four-step process to finding balance with an easy-to-remember acronym, SOUL:

S   Self and spirit (connecting with stress self)

O   Ownership (of life created and how it can be shifted, discovering the mental programming that keeps you stuck and disconnected)

U   Understanding (of the specific path to take)

L   Limitless (possibilities based on path chosen)

For reference, I recommend acquiring a copy of my previous book, *The Mysterious Mind,* which was written to help my patients understand the ancient science of Ayurveda.[6] Although you will still benefit from *The Stress Rx* without it, *The Mysterious Mind* offers helpful supplemental material. It includes quizzes to assess your *dosha* (your Ayurvedic mind-body type, which may be *vata, pitta, or kapha*), and your toxin burden. It has chapters on adrenal fatigue, the gut-brain link (with an emphasis on food intolerances and how to manage them), and a section on lab testing. You'll learn how to evaluate your labs, with your provider, from a functional medicine perspective. This is helpful for those of you who are told "your labs look fine and so are you!" yet know something feels off.

Throughout *The Stress Rx,* footnotes indicate where to find related support material in *The Mysterious Mind.* Resources specific to *The Stress Rx* are available on my website at www.truptigokanimd.com/ stressrxbonus. It has a chapter-by-chapter list linking to each resource noted in *The Stress Rx*. And finally, at the back of *The Stress Rx*, you'll find a glossary of the terms used.

Socrates once said, "An unexamined life is not worth living." I'll take that one step further: I believe an unexamined life prevents you from achieving true health. So, it is my privilege to welcome you to *The Stress Rx*, where we will embark on that examination together and transform your perspective about becoming and remaining healthy. By learning how to change the way you perceive stress, you can take care of 80 to 90 percent of your struggles in your career, your health, your relationships, and all aspects of your life.

Begin by getting to know exactly who you are—how you think, digest, and process your world. Only then can you determine which tools will lead to optimal health for *you*, be it exercise, yoga, or nutrition.

You are meant to be healthy.

1

"Healthy" Is Not What You Think It Is

On a blustery, cold Chicago day in January 1993, I sat in a cozy yet dimly lit therapist's office, exhausted by months of insomnia. As a first-year medical student, sleeplessness impacted me deeply. I could not concentrate or think clearly, so I drifted through my classes and labs in a fog.

I sat quietly on the comfortable green chair facing the therapist's desk as she asked me the following question: "Are you stressed?"

"No, I don't feel stressed," I replied.

Looking back, I realize how little I knew myself at that time or what it truly meant to be healthy and happy. In my early twenties, stress was an unfamiliar concept, and I certainly did not see it as the issue. Insomnia was. I believed stress and insomnia were two very different concerns.

I had hoped a prescription for sleep medication would take me back to my old way of living. Unfortunately, the pills didn't work at the dose prescribed, so I increased the dosage, which led to horrible hangover effects the next day—worse than not sleeping. I stopped the medication. Frustrated and desperate, I told a few trusted souls about my woes, including my parents. Although they did their best to help me, I was disappointed they had no solutions.

I finally reached a point where I couldn't go on. After months without sleeping, and about a month after trying those sleeping pills, I made that visit to the therapist. I explained my struggle with incapacitating insomnia despite attempts to alleviate it with sleeping pills, breathing techniques, and supplements. I had even purchased new bedsheets to perfect the ambiance of my room and bought luxurious, cozy silk pj's for a more comfortable sleep, hoping rest would be restored. Nothing worked. As my roommates slept through the night, I lay awake and stared at the ceiling or wandered through the apartment contemplating ways to navigate my relentless challenge. I was determined to find a solution.

Some of life's challenges, like insomnia, can appear to be insurmountable. We often believe such situations throw us off course. Instead, we might view them as opportunities ultimately intended to get us back on course, not to derail us further. That's what happened to me. The universe would have it no other way.

My bout of insomnia literally woke me up to my life, to the reality of who I was and what I believed. I had been living blindly, following what others had programmed me to believe. Insomnia forced me to look deep inside, to see my truth, and begin living authentically. As my journey unfolded, I began questioning the beliefs I had been programmed to accept—beliefs that did not align with the real me.

I could not see any of this until I began to more deeply explore the question *why is this happening to me?* and shift toward a new question: *what if this is happening* for *me?*

Visiting the therapist initiated my first experience with delving into myself. Turns out, I knew nothing about stress. Because my life appeared good—except for the lack of sleep—I believed I had no reason to feel stress. Thus, I told myself I was not experiencing it. My therapist thought I was fine too, so we had very little to work on.

A month or so later, we parted ways.

Soon after that, I found myself pulling into a psychiatrist's parking lot. As I made my way to his office building, I shivered in the frigid evening temperatures. I had never been to a *shrink,* as they were called in the day, but utter desperation left me with no choice. I was intrigued by this field of medicine and loved learning about the mind. Now, my mind would be analyzed.

As one of my father's most trusted friends, this psychiatrist had my respect. I walked into his small, dark office hoping—and maybe even expecting—he would have the answer to my mysterious ailment. As I took a seat across from his desk, he grabbed a notebook and rattled off questions. Ten minutes and eight questions later, he gave me a diagnosis of depression. He handed me a prescription for Prozac.

Even though I hadn't known what to expect, the brief visit shocked me. I returned to my car in utter despair. Such a quick diagnosis did not make sense. I was not depressed before the onset of insomnia, so how would treating depression get to the root of the problem? Sleeping better would improve my mood, but would improving my mood make me sleep better? The psychiatrist couldn't answer the most intrinsic question: he couldn't tell me the *why* behind my symptoms. His diagnosis simply did not feel right. In that moment, I knew Western tools and diagnostic evaluations weren't addressing my wellness on a deeper level.

As I sat in the driver's seat, shivering from the brisk walk through the parking lot, I pulled the prescription out of my purse and tore it to shreds. That marked the first time in my young adult life that I trusted my inner knowing versus the guidance provided by not only an experienced professional, but also someone I viewed as a father-like figure. Disobeying the psychiatrist, to me, was like disobeying my father.

Until that moment, I had been the good girl who followed the rules. I rarely spoke up. I rarely argued. I obediently listened when told things were to be done a certain way. By tearing up that prescription and not accepting the depression diagnosis, I began trusting my own knowing more than the intelligence of a wise physician. I turned off thoughts of *I should* or *I must* and allowed my inner voice to speak up.

Despite taking that stand, as a first-year medical student, I felt conflicted. How could I continue studying a model of health care that wasn't serving me? I was on the brink of quitting.

Nothing about my situation made sense at that time, yet that is how intuition works. The intuitive voice that told me to rip up the prescription also guided me to a bookstore for answers (before we had the internet). That's where I discovered integrative medicine through the works of Andrew Weil, Deepak Chopra, Bernie Siegel, and eventually, Ayurvedic medicine. My own internal wisdom led me to solutions.

You have that internal wisdom too. It's incredibly powerful. It reflects your truth, your *sat* in Sanskrit. If you are not distracted, you can perceive its fleeting entry into your realm of awareness. With practice, it becomes a silent knowing that you can't necessarily explain, perhaps that churning in your stomach telling you to do or not do something. I am grateful that I was able to hear and act on that wisdom despite being highly distracted—and exhausted—at the time. I can now look back and say insomnia honored me with much-needed pause and reflection. I am truly grateful for the awakening that resulted, as it led me on a path of healing not just for myself but for others as well.

With that awakening, I decided to adjust my perspective from feeling victimized by insomnia to observing it. In doing so, I regained my power. I began to see my situation as a spiritual intervention that forced me to shift my path. Rather than seeking external support with answers from drugs and practitioners, I turned inward to discover myself and the real message behind the insomnia. I continued to spend hours in the bookstore reading self-help publications about mind-body healing and the subtle body—the energy of breath, body, emotions, and thought that influence well-being—taking frequent breaks from my heavy medical reading.

I continuously found answers in the ancient wisdom of Ayurveda, which is believed to be one of the first systems of healing known to humankind. This model and approach opened my eyes to an entirely new way of viewing the mind and body. I realized the emotional body and physical body were one and the same. I learned of the existence of a subtle body, which had equal importance to the physical one, if not more. I finally came to understand the *thinking* brain could block the signaling of the wisdom inherent in all of us. These new understandings inspired a few key lifestyle changes. As part of my insomnia treatment, I began working on the dominant, negative thought patterns that kept me stuck in an endless cycle of sleeplessness. Slowly, powerful outcomes resulted, and sleep returned without medication.

I am grateful for sleeping soundly and having balanced mental health since that time.

Since then, I have also come to realize that my mind had prevented the sleeping pills from being effective. To some degree, I am glad they didn't work. Their failure prompted me to continue the search for answers.

As I continued exploring my innermost self, I looked deeply into Ayurvedic wisdom. It helped me recognize how imbalanced I had been, that my pursuits were disconnected from the truth of how I wanted to live my life. Throughout those early years, when I thought I was healthy, I believed productivity and success came from sustained effort and constant pursuit. There was no time to process or feel emotions. There was no time to rest. I entered the school of medicine knowing it would be taxing, and I felt ready for that. Hard work and long hours didn't frighten me.

Only when my health declined did I awaken to the fallacy of this belief. Working harder is not the answer. Sometimes the most productive thing we can do is to be still. It would take me YEARS to understand that.

DIFFERENT PERSPECTIVES ON HEALTH

Western medicine defines health as the state of being free from illness or injury. By contrast, the Ayurvedic definition of health, in addition to being free of illness or injury, expands to include a strong *agni* (digestive fire) along with balance between the mind, senses, and soul.

Although I barely understood the idea of balance, according to the Ayurvedic definition, I was clearly unhealthy in many ways. I was unhealthy in my habitual thoughts, my negative beliefs, and the way I handled—or did not handle—emotions. I was unhealthy in how I ate, how I exercised, and when I went to sleep. I was unhealthy with the people I allowed in my life, and, of course, I was pursuing my career in an unhealthy manner. These combined aspects of my being led to insomnia. When I finally began tapping into the Ayurvedic wisdom written thousands of years ago, my life forever shifted.

My name, *Trupti*, means "state of being satisfied." Ironically, my life had always been about achievement and wanting more, rarely being satisfied with what I had or had already achieved. Satisfaction, however, can give us so much more peace and happiness than achievements. Although it took half my life to realize this fact, I feel peace knowing we learn what we need to learn in divine time.

The timing of my insomnia could not have been more perfect. As a medical student studying anatomy and histology, I had no preconceived notions about how medicine should be practiced. My father was a physician, yet I had been blessed to rarely need a doctor. Without being locked into a particular way of thinking about health, I was open to other perspectives. Reading books by integrative healers inspired me to learn about health through a much wider lens.

Without question, Western medicine has a place. We are fortunate that it allows us to control severe infections with antibiotics and antivirals, manage acute or chronic pain with highly efficacious tools, and treat malignant tumors with precise regimes of radiation and chemotherapy, as well as offering surgery for conditions ranging from incompetent valves to fractured hips.

Eastern medicine teaches us to look at the body as a messenger that issues warnings, often years before disease sets in. It is imperative we pause when symptoms first begin and seek help, instead of waiting months to years for them to worsen.

WHAT IS HEALTHY?

According to the World Health Organization (WHO), "Health is a state of complete physical, mental, and social well-being and not merely the absence of disease or infirmity."[1] This is more in alignment with the Eastern tradition of Ayurveda than with Western medicine.

Ayurveda defines health—or *swastha*—as encompassing all of who you are:

Health is a state wherein the *tridosha* (constitutional nature), digestive fire, all the body tissues and components, all the physiological processes are in perfect unison and the soul, the sense organs, and the mind are in a state of total satisfaction and contentment.

As you can see, *healthy* is more than a well-functioning body. A healthy person is defined as:

One who is established in self, who has balanced doshas, balanced agni, properly formed *dhatus* (body tissues), proper elimination of *malas* (wastes), well-functioning bodily processes, and whose mind, soul, and senses are happy is called a healthy person.

You can achieve this balance of mind, body, and spirit through holistic medicine, by taking the time to honor your symptoms when they arise. Addressing them earlier rather than later reduces the burden of disease and the cost of health care.

In the early to mid-seventeenth century, philosophers such as René Descartes shared the gospel of "I think, therefore I am," believing that the mind is separate from the body. This was later debated by neuroscientists such as Antonio Damasio, who called such observations an error. Damasio even wrote a book on the topic, sharing his idea that thinking requires guidance from emotions and feelings, which are conveyed by the body.[2] In fact, research shows that the physiological state of the gut microbiome dictates how we feel and process stress—and thus how we think![3]

The public began to question whether the mind and body operated independently or in unison. This is exactly in alignment with Ayurvedic wisdom taught over five thousand years ago.

MIND, BODY, OR SPIRIT: WHAT'S IN CONTROL?

You may be wondering . . . does the mind control the body?

Or does the body influence the mind?

Mind, body, and spiritual health are enigmatic conversations for most. Many are unsure if religion or spirituality should be included as part of a health care discussion. Due to this debate, in 1802 at the end of the French Revolution, medicine and religion were officially separated. These days, however, increasing evidence suggests that adding a spiritual component to health care may lead to improved longevity.[4] It may also lead to a reduction in inflammatory cytokines.[5]

The purely medical model gave me a diagnosis and prescription, which left me feeling unheard and misunderstood. While I tried to explain the sleep challenges and my curiosity regarding the onset, the physician wanted me to align with a "checklist" of symptoms for a specific diagnosis, and thus, a precise remedy. I only wish it were that simple: one drug working on one neurotransmitter fixing a complex issue. But we are intricate human beings who rarely present with simple conditions. At that time, I sought a deeper answer reflecting on the health of my mind, my senses, and my spiritual self.

When insomnia first struck, my Western primary care physician gave me a physical exam and ordered blood tests. Because everything indicated I was "normal," he told me there was nothing wrong with me. The therapist had nothing to offer either, since I didn't appear stressed, and my moods seemed fine to her. Yet there *was* something wrong with me. It resided at a deeper level of my system, in an area not recognized by routine testing or evaluations.

Studies reveal that 60 to 90 percent of office visits to the primary care provider are due to stress-related conditions.[6] Yet besides the one therapist asking whether I suffered from stress, there was very little discussion about how stress led to the manifestation of my sleep challenges. Since I was not aware how stress manifested, I believed that stress was not part of my condition.

As I look back, it is fascinating to me that we ask others outside of ourselves to give us a perspective on our well-being—like me, turning to the therapist, who asked if I felt stressed. But when we are in a stressed state (which was twenty-four seven for me as a medical student), how do you even know what it feels like to *not* be stressed? I was driven for most of my life. I even won an award in sixth grade as the "hardest worker in the class." Hard work was all I knew. That had become my persona, and I didn't recognize stress as a part of it.

The beauty of Ayurveda is that it provides a perspective on how disconnected we are from our most ideal, harmonious self.

In my early twenties, my driven personality allowed me to survive some challenging times. Continuing to live that way became self-destructive. Since our bodily systems want nothing but for us to be safe, and the many pressures of my life at that time did not subconsciously *feel* safe, my brain instructed me to stay awake and be alert for danger coming my way. My physiology shifted and then led to troubled nights of sleep.

This particular danger-state eventually taxes the adrenal system. *The Mysterious Mind* devotes an entire chapter to adrenal fatigue.** Not so long ago, Western medicine was skeptical of adrenal fatigue, so I began studying my clinic patients to prove that it existed. Eventually, I stopped testing for it, as 90 percent of my patients exhibited symptoms: sugar cravings, digestion issues, inability to handle stress, low moods,

---

* Read more about this and the different phases of the stress response in *The Mysterious Mind*, chapter 6, "Adrenal Fatigue: A Hidden Pervasive Syndrome."

dizziness, forgetfulness, brain fog, overwhelm, sluggishness, and, despite the sluggishness, a continual urge to move.

Western medicine has come to recognize these symptoms as hypothalamic-pituitary-adrenal maladaptation syndrome. Yes, a mouthful. Let's call it HPA maladaptation syndrome. It is now understood that adrenal fatigue—a.k.a. HPA maladaptation syndrome—is more of a brain problem than an adrenal problem, as once believed.

The Stress Rx explores various tools to reconnect with yourself and alleviate the harmful effects of stress. Engaging with the exercises to come will allow you to find your state of bliss. It exists, I promise.

A NEW MODEL FOR HEALTH

Feeling misaligned with the major depression diagnosis drove me to search for another verdict. After reading Ayurvedic textbooks and learning as much as I could on the topic, I determined that I was in *vata* imbalance, eventually leading to *vata-pitta* imbalance. Vata is one of the three mind-body types in Ayurveda (pitta is another). I had an excess of this nature, which led to my initial issues with falling asleep.

The Eastern diagnosis refers to the *subtle body*—or energy. The subtle body embodies thoughts, emotions, wisdom, and life force energy, which all link to breath. This is how connecting with your breath and regulating it helps cope with tension and stress. The subtle body is one of the most crucial aspects of your being. A thorough understanding of it must be incorporated into an exploration of health.

Currently, conventional approaches do not address the subtle body. To move beyond the current medical crisis, our health care systems must abandon their narrow view of health and consider mind, body, and spirit for total health. This is the focus of *The Stress Rx*.

Over the last two decades, I have watched thousands of patients transform their health by utilizing this model. It addresses stress by using ancient wisdom to evaluate and connect with the subtle body. As it surely becomes clear, the ignored subtle body leads to stress, eventually manifesting as disease.

The current health care model prevents you from achieving health by focusing on the physical body; limiting conversations about the connections between mental, emotional, and spiritual health; and ignoring the gut-brain link from an energetic perspective.

By relying upon the Western model alone—by not addressing these limitations—challenges to preventing and combating disease will remain. The time has come to incorporate a more integrated approach to health that embraces the wisdom of ancient medicine.

I believe we are ready for this.

TAKE-HOME POINTS

1. Shifting from *why is this happening to me?* toward a new question, *what if this is happening* for *me?* is a powerful way to evaluate a challenging time and grow from it.

2. The *thinking* brain, especially when stuck in negative thought patterns, can block the signaling of the wisdom (intuition) inherent in all of us.

3. The Western definition of health is limited to being free of illness or injury. The Ayurvedic definition of health expands to include a strong agni (digestive fire) along with balance between the mind, senses, and soul.

4. Studies reveal that 60 to 90 percent of office visits to the primary care provider are due to stress-related conditions.

5. Ayurveda shows us how disconnected we are from our most ideal, harmonious self.

6. The Eastern diagnosis refers to the subtle body, which embodies the mind, along with the spiritual and social well-being aspect

of your health. The subtle body embodies your thoughts, emotions, wisdom, and life force energy, which are all linked to your breath.

7. The subtle body is just as important for health as the physical body—if not more so.

SELF-CARE TIME

Take the stress personality quiz, available through www.truptigokanimd.com/stressrxbonus. This will help you understand how far you are from alignment and optimal health.

Why should you do this?

If you avoid getting to know yourself first, you won't be equipped to make choices that align with your true self. Your choices may further pull your life out of balance, eventually leading to poor health, disease, increased doctor's visits, and lower quality of life. If you long to finally shift your health for the better, keep reading. To be healthy, happy, and prosperous, we must evaluate ourselves, specifically our subtle body. Over time, the burden of disease may lead to struggles with family, significant others, and work. We may lose friends or even a career due to health struggles. We are also at risk of raising kids who perpetuate the burden of imbalance. As we work on ourselves, we indirectly work on their imbalances too.

How great is that gift as a parent?

The reason one becomes stressed, overwhelmed, and unhealthy is not that one is not trying. It is because one has not taken the time to get to know oneself. Once this is accomplished, it becomes easy to figure out the best approach for becoming healthy, happy, and strong.

The path is scripted in ancient medicine.

Let us start the journey!

2

Resolving the Conflict Within

"Nobody can bring peace but yourself."
—Ralph Waldo Emerson

During the mythical battle in the land of Kurukshetra, the mighty warrior Arjuna lays down his arms in a moment of confusion. This powerful scene appears in the Bhagavad Gita, one of the most revered texts on ancient wisdom. With 701 verses and originally written in Sanskrit, the Bhagavad Gita has been translated into English hundreds of times since the eighteenth century due to its powerful message.

In the scene described above, Arjuna entered a battle against his own family, a battle between good and evil. Yet Arjuna was tormented by the idea of potentially killing those he loved, even though they represented unjust and malicious thoughts and actions. He stood with one side of his family for their beliefs and values. They had tried to resolve the conflict without fighting those who held opposing views and reached a point where they were left with no choice.

Arjuna's wise guide, Krishna, sat in the chariot as Arjuna's mentor to help him discover how to proceed. The answer was seeded deeply within Arjuna, clouded by his distracted and confused mind. To find a solution, Arjuna had to align his inner truth with his sense of duty and act according to his highest self. For as much as the conflict appeared to be on the outside, it was truly an internal battle.

This scene in the Gita represents the most fundamental core to thriving in life. It is the message of how to orchestrate the battle within. Like Arjuna, our battles may appear external, but the truth is they stem from internal struggles that eventually manifest on the outside.

Over the many years I have been working on myself, along with helping others achieve success in health, relationships, and their careers, I realized that the first step in improving life is to pause and reflect on internal battles. Evaluating them can help you understand the challenges surrounding you on the outside. As difficult as it may seem, it is the first step to creating balance in mind, body, and spirit.

So how do you accomplish this? Where do you even begin?

In chapter 1, you had the opportunity to take the stress personality type quiz.[1] I developed this quiz after years of studying Ayurveda and applying it to real life. Many patients, clients, family members, and friends shared their pain, anxiety, and dissatisfaction with life. Even though their basic needs for food and shelter were met or even exceeded—and most lived comfortably—they were still unhappy. A common theme emerged. Whether they experienced migraines, hair loss, or difficulty sleeping, there was a disconnect between their inner and outer worlds, and Western tools were simply not helping enough.

You may not be ready to delve into the lofty *whys* behind your symptoms, especially if some basic core needs are not being met. For example, if you struggle with migraines and are challenged with cycles of pain that are not responsive to medications, then your focus will be on the pain and how to eradicate it. This means, for most, you will focus on your core survival needs first, and ONLY when those needs are satisfied will you have the energy to dig into your whys. Understanding this, I realized how important it was to control the pain with safe and effective tools. In the case of those struggling with migraines, the first step was ensuring they had what they needed to abort the pain and function. Then, we could move on to deeper conversations and reflect on why the pain appeared in the first place.

Abraham Maslow's hierarchy of needs best illustrates this concept. Although Maslow's theory has encountered some criticism over its less-than-scientific approach, it shares good insight into human motivation. As illustrated in figure 2.1, specific, immediate needs must be met first. Once individuals have fresh air, water, food, and shelter, they can evolve toward higher needs, first for self, then family, then the world.

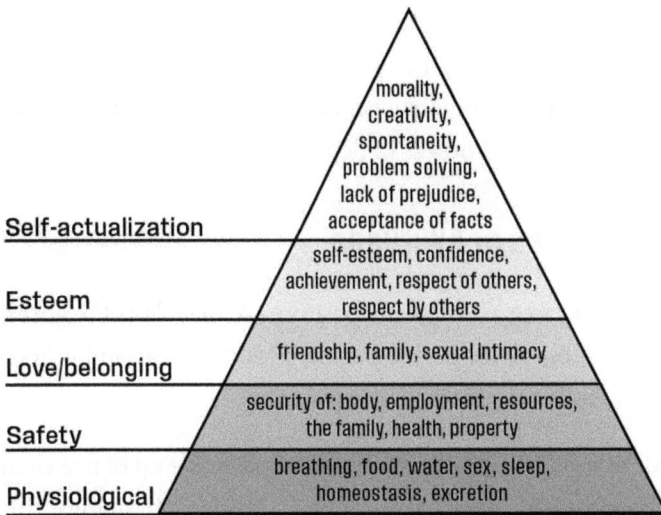

Self-actualization — morality, creativity, spontaneity, problem solving, lack of prejudice, acceptance of facts

Esteem — self-esteem, confidence, achievement, respect of others, respect by others

Love/belonging — friendship, family, sexual intimacy

Safety — security of: body, employment, resources, the family, health, property

Physiological — breathing, food, water, sex, sleep, homeostasis, excretion

MAZLOW'S HIERARCHY OF NEEDS

Maslow's Hierarchy of Needs[2]

AYURVEDA AND CONNECTING WITH SELF

Delving into a current conflict is one of the best ways to evaluate internal battles. Everyone, at some level, has inner conflict. It may be minor, such as debating whether Mexican or Italian food wins for dinner. At other times, the conflict may be major, such as wondering if your job of twenty years still aligns with your values and goals. When someone is conflicted or struggling with internal battles, they begin moving out of alignment.

After my self-guided study of Ayurveda in my early twenties, I realized just how out of alignment and disconnected I was. Since I had been living in that state for so long, I was too unaware to recognize it on my own. Sometimes it takes an outside observer to reveal our truth. This is what Ayurveda did for me. By allowing me to delve into my inner nature through various Ayurvedic quizzes, I quickly discovered why I was struggling so much. Even though the doctors told me I was healthy, according to Ayurveda, I was not.

As unique as each of you are in your journey and struggle, take some comfort in knowing that we humans share profound similarities. Whether balanced or imbalanced, our state of being will have certain elements in excess and others in depletion.

Basic Principles of Ayurveda

Ayur means life and *veda* means wisdom. Ayurveda is the wisdom of life or the wisdom of longevity. Dating back five thousand years, it has specific principles as part of its framework:

1. All things, inanimate and animate, are made up of five elements: air, space, fire, earth, and water. In human physiology, this creates your mind-body energy type known as your dosha.

2. At birth, you are in your most aligned state. This is known as your *prakruti*, your birth nature or constitutional state. Your elemental makeup at birth is considered to be your authentic state.

3. During life, you become imbalanced as you choose careers, friends, significant others, food, and lifestyles that push your elements out of alignment. This leads to an imbalanced state known as *vikruti*.

4. The goal is to shift your lifestyle, foods, friends, career, etc. so you can move from imbalanced vikruti to balanced prakruti. (Easier said than done. Believe me, I know.)

5. When symptoms occur, even if they begin subtly and mildly, consider them a warning that you are out of alignment. The initial imbalance may simply be a feeling of being off. You may have problems focusing, low energy, difficulty with tasks, experience gut issues, or even problems sleeping. You may find that your moods are difficult to control. The symptoms provide a clue to which system needs some balancing. These are the first signs of stress on the system.

6. Disease occurs when you have lived out of alignment for too long.

7. Food, especially spices, are considered medicinal, and thus used to heal.

8. The mind and body are one. What you think, you are, and vice versa. If you think negative thoughts, your body will hold negative vibrations, leading to an imbalanced physiology.

9. Ayurveda and yoga are sister sciences. Incorporating the mind, breathwork, and physical *asanas* (poses) of yoga, along with knowledge of your Ayurvedic imbalance, gives you powerful tools to create health, happiness, and prosperity in all areas of life.

CONNECTION & DISCONNECTION:

Connection to Self, Authentic Nature Leads to Balance
Disconnection from Self = Stress - Leads to State Imbalance

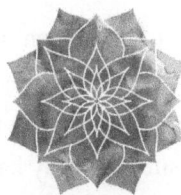
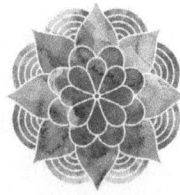

Vata   Pitta   Kapha

Stress Won't Let You Be You

Practicing Ayurveda creates an optimal and balanced state. In this state, you become focused, energetic, and free of symptoms. Maintaining optimal performance is challenging. It requires close attention to yourself and your situation. Demands of your external world and internal programs can easily pull you into low- or high-stress states.

Figure 2.3 contrasts the optimal performance state with impacts on performance and the mind during low and high periods of stress. It is not a pretty picture!

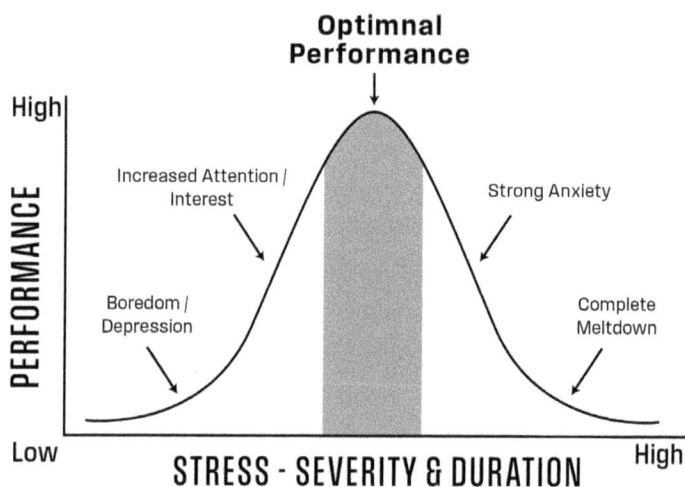

THE STRESS PERSONALITY STATE

As I mentioned earlier, each of us is born into prakruti, or a balanced energy state. Were we to live without stress, we might remain there. However, life rarely works that way. If you took the stress personality type quiz found on my website, you may have discovered that instead of balanced, your personality has become overly fiery, windy, or earthy.

You are probably wondering how you got there.

Unfortunately, moving out of alignment is common. The world naturally provokes imbalance. Without proactively caring for yourself, you will easily move into disharmony. For example, your approach to life is out of balance when your behavior ignores your circadian rhythm. You might go to bed late because you worked late and needed some time to unwind before falling sleep. Perhaps you engage in multitasking to accomplish more and skip breaks or meals because you're in a rush. In addition, eating foods your body type doesn't easily process—like those convenient fast foods—leads to disharmony. Repeated over time, each of these actions slowly shifts you out of your prakruti.

Disconnection begins with a shift in the subtle body, which is the energy behind your thoughts, emotions, wisdom, and prana or life force energy. Then, the physical system starts to present imbalance. These changes occur in an insidious fashion. Early on, you may not be aware of your subtle body shifting. But before you know it, symptoms appear. You may feel more anxious or worried. You may feel sad for no apparent reason. You may struggle with falling or staying asleep, or your digestion may feel off.

The mind-body type, or the dosha, becomes vitiated (imbalanced) leading to excess vata, pitta, or kapha energy. An excess of one dosha happens at the expense of the other doshas. This shift in the subtle body often occurs before the physical body manifests the change. Often, one dosha is high while another is low.

Dosha Types

Vata

Dosha: Vata

Element: Windy

Qualities: Elements of air and space and characterized by movement, dryness, and lightness

Physical Symptoms of Imbalance: Dry skin and hair, constipation or irregular bowel movements, joint pain or stiffness, weight loss, insomnia or disturbed sleep, irregular menstrual cycles.

Mental/Emotional: Symptoms of Imbalance: Anxiety or excessive worry, restlessness or inability to focus, fear or nervousness, overwhelm or feeling scattered.

Pitta

Dosha: Pitta

Element: Fiery

Qualities: Elements of fire and water, characterized by heat, sharpness, and intensity.

Physical Symptoms of Imbalance: acid reflux, heartburn, loose stools, migraine headaches, skin rashes, excessive hunger or body heat.

Kapha

Dosha: Kapha

Element: Earthy

Qualities: Elements of earth and water, characterized by heaviness, stability, and moisture

Physical Symptoms of Imbalance: Weight gain or difficulty losing weight, lethargy or sluggishness, excess mucus production (e.g., congestion, sinus issues), water retention or swelling, oily skin or hair, slow digestion or feeling heavy after eating.

Mental/Emotional: Symptoms of Imbalance: Depression or lack of motivation, attachment or resistance to change, greed or possessiveness, over-sentimentality or holding onto the past.

The five elements—air, space, fire, earth, and water—create our mind, body, and spirit. When some elements are in higher proportion due to life factors such as diet, lifestyle, or stress, then the other elements are reduced. In the disconnected state, you may not even realize that you are in the thick of it; you are not able to see the forest for the trees. You must step away from the imbalanced state long enough to gain perspective. It's like trying on a new pair of glasses with a more accurate prescription. Suddenly, you can see. Until you wore the new glasses, you did not realize the depth of your impaired vision.

My experience with the therapist so many years ago was like that. When asked if I was stressed, I said no. I couldn't see the forest for the trees. I was in the thick of it.

Your subtle body operates in the same way. Most people do not realize it is imbalanced. Yet once you tap into it and begin to observe and strengthen it, everything changes. You cannot unsee what you have seen. Clarity emerges regarding yourself and your being. You don't realize how bad you feel until you start feeling good. You do not want to experience the unbalanced state again.

So, why do you go out of state (become imbalanced), and why do you stay there?

THE BRAIN AND NERVOUS SYSTEM

Let's take a moment to review how your system operates with a high-level overview of the brain and nervous system. (No quiz at the end, I promise!) The more you understand about your brain, the easier it will be to understand the approaches used to balance it.

Through his concept of the triune brain, Paul MacLean organized the human brain into three distinct regions:

1. The Neomammalian or Neocortex

   More commonly known as the prefrontal cortex, or PFC, this is the thinking, rational brain. It allows us to perform higher-level thinking, analysis, and discernment. When the PFC is active and the right and left hemispheres are balanced, humans think about situations in a multifaceted way. We become more open and receptive to different perspectives, thoughts, and ideas.

The PFC helps us to organize ourselves and perform executive functions such as utilizing working memory, flexible thinking, and self-control. With this part of the nervous system engaged and active, we can feel compassion, love, joy, and bliss, as
well as happiness for others and for ourselves. This part of the
brain allows us to be self-aware and express ourselves verbally.

In humans, the PFC does not fully develop until the age of
twenty-five, which explains some of the unpredictable behavior
witnessed in teenagers. In fact, in her early teens, my brilliant
daughter would say to me, "Mom, don't expect me to behave. My
PFC is still not fully developed!"[3]

2. The Mammalian Brain or Limbic Brain

This is the "feeling" brain. It allows us to process and express
emotion. Consider it to be the home for your emotional baggage. Memories and experiences become trapped in the amygdala, a key structure of the limbic brain, if we do not take the
time to process and clear them.

About 90 percent of human operations happen at a subconscious level. The amygdala plays a big role in perceiving and responding to threats—even before we are consciously aware of
them. It receives sensory input from the five senses through the
thalamus gland and from the olfactory nerve directly. When it
perceives danger, the amygdala alerts the hypothalamus to activate the sympathetic nervous system (SNS), initiating the fight-
or-flight response, which then turns on your adrenal glands to
make stress hormones.

Recent science has found the ENS—the nervous system
in the gut—is a peripheral extension of the limbic brain. That
means the limbic, feeling brain extends itself into the gut. This
is probably why we have "gut feelings" or a "gut instinct" about
something.[4]

3. The Reptilian Brain/Basal Ganglia

Also known as the "survival" brain or reptilian brain, the basal ganglia is the system in the brain similar to that of reptiles and is believed to focus on self-preservation. It protects us from danger. It is linked to the brainstem and centers on heart rate, respiration, digestion, alertness, and core nervous system functions.

Our instinctive, reflexive responses come from the reptilian brain. These responses do not engage the higher-level neocortex for processing. When the reptilian brain is activated, we simply react without thinking; the goal of survival takes over.

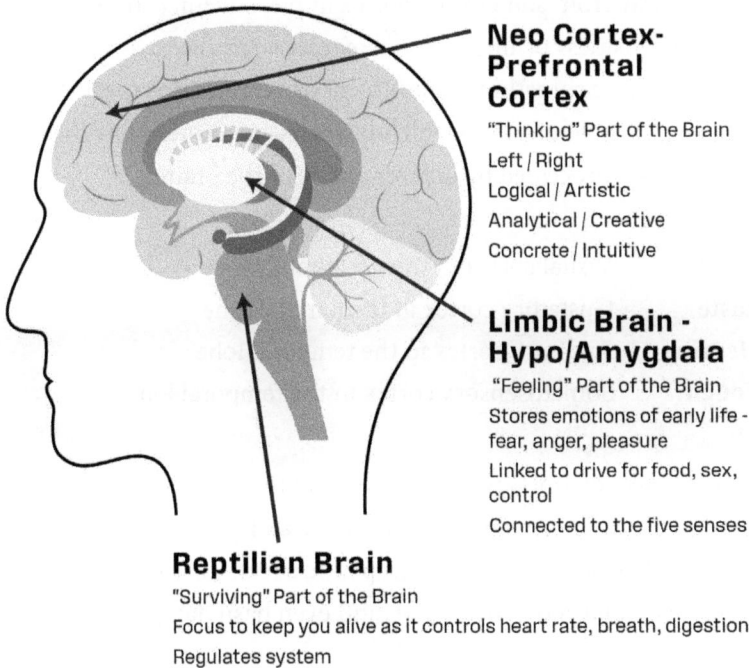

**Neo Cortex-
Prefrontal
Cortex**
"Thinking" Part of the Brain
Left / Right
Logical / Artistic
Analytical / Creative
Concrete / Intuitive

**Limbic Brain -
Hypo/Amygdala**
"Feeling" Part of the Brain
Stores emotions of early life -
fear, anger, pleasure
Linked to drive for food, sex,
control
Connected to the five senses

Reptilian Brain
"Surviving" Part of the Brain
Focus to keep you alive as it controls heart rate, breath, digestion
Regulates system

Within the limbic brain, the hypothalamus operates as a circadian pacemaker, regulating appetite centers, body temperature, breathing rate, heartbeat, and other core functions of the reptilian brain. I call it the divine internal mother (or father). It receives information from other parts of the brain—the amygdala, for example—and then determines which hormones or neurotransmitters to release. The signal for release is sent through the pituitary gland, the master gland regulating hormones.

Sensing Temptation

Our five senses—sight, taste, hearing, touch, and smell—tempt us in different ways. The sense of taste may compel us to eat that extra slice of pizza, even when we are full. The sense of sight may prompt Netflix binging. Senses continually stimulate us.

Senses connect to our desires. At times, they may turn us off or draw us away from something. For example, smelling something that triggers queasiness or uneasiness may cause appetite loss or a change of mood. Seeing something reminiscent of a traumatic experience may prompt anxiety. Four senses—all but smell—are captured by the thalamus and then processed by different parts of the brain.

Sight	Visual cortex in the occipital lobe
Taste	Gustatory cortex in the parietal lobe
Hearing	Auditory cortex in the temporal lobe
Touch	Somatosensory cortex in the temporal lobe

The sense of smell is unique; it is captured directly by olfactory receptors in the nose. Smell has a direct and powerful effect on the amygdala that can be used for therapeutic effect. Calming and relaxing scents such as lavender, bergamot, and even basil dampen its activity.

OTHER PARTS OF THE NERVOUS SYSTEM

The reticular activating system (RAS) is located above the spinal cord, where it registers sensory input from all senses except smell. It filters information and activates the PFC based on what is deemed significant. It helps direct attention to what your mind feels is important.

The RAS and other brain regions, such as the anterior cingulate cortex (ACC), help mobilize the PFC, the limbic, or the reptilian brain based on your unique brain program. Modifying your program through Ayurveda can strengthen these areas so they do not overly arouse the limbic and reptilian brains to perceived danger.

The PFC should activate when you want to perform higher-level functions such as thinking, making decisions, having conversations, and observing or listening. The limbic brain should activate when an emotional situation arises so you can tap into your emotional body to assist yourself or others. The reptilian brain, while always active and on alert for your protection, should only take the lead in times of acute stress. Problems occur when too many perceived stressors arise during the day or when stressful feelings persist after the situation has been resolved. Acute stress then becomes chronic, persistent, and pervasive.*

When stress shifts from acute to chronic, balance between the three brain areas is exchanged for dominance in the limbic or reptilian brain. Reactions and thinking become more reptilian. In this state, people are triggered easily and have a hard time settling down. This leads to a spiraling cycle of emotional overload and a reduced ability to respond appropriately.

When the RAS or ACC are not filtering incoming cues appropriately, the limbic brain or its extension in the gut, the ENS, become overly activated. Overactivation hijacks the PFC from thinking clearly. Instead of controlling the limbic brain and ENS, those areas run the show and trigger the stress-response system. The reptilian brain takes over, viewing the world as dangerous. The reptilian brain goes into dominance, creating internal conflict and heightening stress levels further. When this happens, we function more like our reptilian

---

* Read more about this and the different phases of the stress response in *The Mysterious Mind*, chapter 6, "Adrenal Fatigue: A Hidden Pervasive Syndrome."

friends—becoming angry and reactive, for example—and we behave less like balanced and calm humans.

Internal conflict yields external conflict.

The peripheral nervous system, the PNS, is an extension of the brain and spinal cord. It consists of nerves and nerve bundles forming the network of communication between the brain and spinal cord with the body and organs to maintain cohesive operations.

The PNS is made up of the somatic and autonomic nervous systems. The somatic nervous system regulates voluntary muscle function. The autonomic nervous system (ANS) regulates involuntary functions.

Let's take a closer look at the automatic nervous system. Most believe that the ANS is made up of two parts, the sympathetic and the parasympathetic nervous systems (SNS and ParaNS, respectively). Some thinkers believe there is a third part, the ENS mentioned earlier.

The SNS, sympathetic nervous system, functions to mobilize resources. It maintains alertness so we can attend to our needs. With the help of the stress hormone cortisol, this system allows us to wake up and take care of tasks. When under duress, it creates the fight, flight, or freeze response to protect us from impending or perceived danger.

The ParaNS serves to conserve resources. This system, when turned on, allows us to replenish the body or reset after being taxed and depleted.

The ENS is believed by some brilliant researchers, such as Dr. Michael Gershon, who wrote the book *The Second Brain*, to be the third part of the ANS.[5] This is the intricate and complex nervous system that lies within the gut. As stated above, the ENS is believed to be the peripheral extension of the limbic brain.

We have twelve nerves dedicated to the brain in our head. The vagus nerve connects the gut and the brain. Breathing deeply and engaging the diaphragm activates the vagus and quiets the mind. This step offers a simple approach to establishing equilibrium between the stress personality and the imbalanced energy state known as vikruti.

Vagus means the fugitive, the wanderer, or the roving nerve. We call it the "busybody" because it has to be involved in everything! The longest cranial nerve in the body, it engages with every bodily system to provide the brain with input about what is going on in your body. The vagus nerve creates a powerful connection between the gut and the brain. Incredibly, more conversation travels from the gut to the brain than from the brain to the gut.

WHAT?

Your gut tells you more about your system than your brain does? Absolutely!

Eighty percent of the vagal nerve's work is sensory. It reports activity of the viscera—end organs such as the gut, heart, and lungs—back to the brain. As I said earlier, it is the busybody-wanderer, giving the brain the scoop about all the body's organs.

Before we take a closer look at what drives you into an imbalanced state and how to move back into harmony, let's quickly review the main points of this chapter and look at a few action steps you can take to put what you've learned to work.

TAKE-HOME POINTS:

1. Internal conflict leads to external challenges.

2. Ayurveda is a five-thousand-year-old science based on the principle that all living beings are composed of five elements: air, space, fire, earth, and water.

3. You are most balanced at birth. Life pulls you out of balance.

4. Understanding how you have disconnected from your authentic state is the key to resolving your inner conflict.

5. The brain has three main areas: the prefrontal cortex (PFC), limbic brain (ENS), and reptilian brain.

6. Your five senses, with the help of the reticular activating system (RAS) and the anterior cingulate cortex (ACC), stimulate higher

brain function (PFC) with control of your lower brain (ENS). When stress levels run too high or linger for too long, your reptilian takes over.

7. For total health, all parts of your brain physiology must operate in a balanced fashion. If one area dominates the others, internal conflict results.

8. The parasympathetic nervous system (ParaNS, your rest-and-relax system), and sympathetic nervous system (SNS, your fight-or flight-system), are part of the ANS nervous system, along with the ENS.

9. The vagus nerve connects the ENS and gut directly to the brain.

10. More messages come from the gut to the brain than from the brain to the gut.

SELF-CARE TIME

To take the most effective initial step toward resolving the conflict within you, get in touch with where you are now and clearly establish where you want to go. Grab a journal and free-flow your responses to the suggestions below.

- What are your current challenges? Where are your conflicts?
- In which area of life do they occur: family, relationships, health, career . . . or all four?
- How would you describe your battle?
- Choose one area of conflict and reflect upon it.
- Reflect upon your stress personality type. How does that relate to your conflicts?
- Ponder which experiences allowed you to move into that imbalanced state.

3

The Forgotten Body
(or the Not-So-Subtle Body)

"Be responsible for the energy you bring into the room."
A friend said those words to me as we entered the conference room
for a mastermind training session with some of the most highly re-
spected clinicians at that time. I had a faint idea of what she was talking
about, yet I was not entirely sure how to achieve it. As an avid yogini
in my early forties, I was still grappling with the idea that our bodies
are composed of more empty space than matter, and that humans are
spiritual beings living a physical experience.

Discoveries accumulated from my own personal journey and from
witnessing my patients' experiences drew me forward, and now, after
years of training in energy medicine, I finally appreciate the meaning
of my friend's powerful words. Each one of us is capable of regulating
and aligning with our most highly tuned selves, and thus, we bear responsibility for the energy we exude, for the type of presence we bring
into a room.

How do we reach a vibrant, high-energy state?

The key is clearing out the parts of yourself that hold you back
from being fully vibrant. In simpler terms, you need to get rid of your
baggage. That, my friends, is our biggest challenge.

In Ayurveda, we call that baggage *ama*. Ama can be referred to as a dangerous toxin. Toxins are not only physical; they are also emotional. You become toxic when you hold onto the emotions of experiences and attitudes that do not serve you.

Let me take you back to the concept of conflict. Remember that any inner conflict leads to external conflict, blocking access to a harmonious state. A blocked internal state, which creates internal ama, leads to a blocked external state, thus preventing you from achieving the health, prosperity, and abundance you so dream of.

Simply put, inner conflict leads to a rise in your internal ama, which then prevents you from being in tune with your highest self. Once people understand they are out of alignment in one or more areas of their lives, they want to find that ama and clear it as quickly as possible.

Now that you understand your neurology at a deeper level, let's dig into the part of the nervous system that most people dare not go. Most of you are comfortable discussing your physical body. You know what pain to your physical body looks like. You may look at yourself in the mirror in the morning and think you look flushed or ill, your hair is a mess, or your outfit doesn't suit you. You are all well-versed in evaluating your physical state.

Yet are you able to assess your subtle or energetic state? That's where the ama lingers.

I spent years studying structures of the brain and the nervous system. As you are now aware, this system allows humans to mobilize, engage in conversation, and perform higher-level functions as a human. Most people, and their medical service providers, have a hard time evaluating anything more than the physical presentation of symptoms. They don't take into account the thought processes, emotions, intuition, and life force energy of the subtle body. I often refer to the subtle body as the forgotten body simply because most practitioners forget that it even exists—or never learned that it exists in the first place.

Not only does the subtle body exist, it also plays an incredibly important role in human well-being. In fact, its influence on overall health is more powerful than the physical itself.

MEET YOUR SUBTLE BODY

When I discuss subtle energy, let me clarify: simply because I say it is *subtle* doesn't mean it is less powerful. In fact, it is the most powerful aspect of your being. This is where I lose most people, so please bear with me, as this is the missing piece of the health puzzle, the part that most Westerners ignore. The subtle body represents your energy and life force, so let's begin by exploring the subtle body in terms of energy. Many of you frequently use the word *energy* in your conversations. Common expressions include:

I am feeling energetic today.

Her energy is amazing!

I need an energy boost.

This house has bad energy!

Most people believe that to increase your energy, you must consume something such as energy drinks—including coffee—or energy supplements or work out. Unfortunately, most quick fixes do not impact the subtle energy system I am referring to. In fact, over the long term, most of them deplete the energy body.

WHAT IS ENERGY?

The *Merriam-Webster Dictionary* defines energy in several ways. This definition partly describes what we're talking about:

> Energy is a fundamental entity of nature that is transferred between parts of a system in the production of physical change within the system and is usually regarded as the capacity for doing work.[1]

A few other definitions include: "Vigorous exertion of power (effort)" and "a usually positive spiritual force."[2]

Whoa . . . *spiritual*?

When did energy become spiritual? What does that even mean?

Those questions lead to a complicated conversation for sure. I'll save that part of the conversation for later, but you can see why the discussion of human energy might become challenging. This is especially true when I raise it with a group of physicians and health care providers at medical conferences, because my kind and well-intentioned academic colleagues prefer to discuss objective and tangible elements of health. If it hadn't been for my quest to solve my insomnia challenge, and the feeling I had no choice but to move beyond the physical body for answers, I might feel as they do. But when my sleep issues weren't resolved by addressing diet, magnesium intake, uncomfortable bedding, a too-warm room temperature, or medication, Ayurveda led me to the subtle body—my energy life force—as the cause of the imbalance. That's where I found my solution. That doesn't mean there weren't any physical components to my insomnia, but it does mean they played a smaller role than traditional Western medicine might suggest.

Within my energy body, I discovered layers of ama that needed cleansing. Some of the ama was physical, due to excess gluten and dairy intake. A larger portion of the ama was mental, resulting from the negative thoughts and programs I carried about myself and my life.

When I ripped up my Prozac prescription after visiting a well-meaning psychiatrist, I knew there was another direction for me. I had no idea what that direction might be, but I felt certain something was missing. Remember, at that moment, I knew nothing about mind-body medicine and Ayurveda. All I had been exposed to was the Western model.

Since then, I've met patients from all walks of life who tried to fix their physical bodies by exercising, changing their diet, taking supplements, and even getting surgery to correct structural issues. In the end, many of them reported that although symptoms improved initially, they never fully resolved. In some cases, they even worsened. Their experience prompted me to add energy medicine to my practice. I help my patients recognize the importance of the subtle body—of the thoughts, emotions, and breath that contribute to their life force energy.

My first book, *The Mysterious Mind,* focused on migraine head-aches, a common and pervasive symptom of many imbalances. Migraine and pain disorders are subjective, not objective. As such, they are difficult for Western health care systems to deal with. People who experience migraines may describe the unique phenomena of flickering lights, numbness, sensitivities to light and sound, pulsating head pain, and vertigo, yet a physical exam and an MRI scan will indicate everything is normal. In fact, migraine is the routine diagnosis of such symptoms when all the testing and exams appear normal. Some higher-level diagnostic tests may point to shifts in glucose utilization, blood flow, or electrical activity in parts of the brain where the pain is felt or perceived, yet the effect is temporary and usually not due to structural issues.

Pain exists, yet it can rarely be measured beyond one's subjective interpretation. This is quite a problem for the Western world, where we want to see it to believe it. We want abnormal imaging reports or lab results for objective proof that pain exists.

What happens when no abnormalities are found in the testing, when you are told you are fine even though you do not feel fine? In such cases, the subtle body is involved. Because the majority of your health care providers haven't been trained in the subtle body, they can only report you are "fine" or "normal," or worse, they'll tell you it's all in your head.

It's not in your head; it's in your subtle body.

YOUR KOSHAS

To further define the subtle body, I will refer to the *koshas,* known in yoga as the sheaths or the layers that make up your subtle body and the essence of who you are. The outermost sheath is the *annamaya kosha* (the physical body layer). Working inward from the annamaya kosha lies the *pranamaya kosha* (breath layer), the *manomaya kosha* (mind layer), the *vijnanamaya kosha* (intellect layer), and at the core, the *anandamaya kosha* (bliss layer). Together, these sheaths or layers comprise your subtle energy body and the essence of your being.

Balancing the koshas is linked to alignment of the chakras, which we discuss later in this chapter.

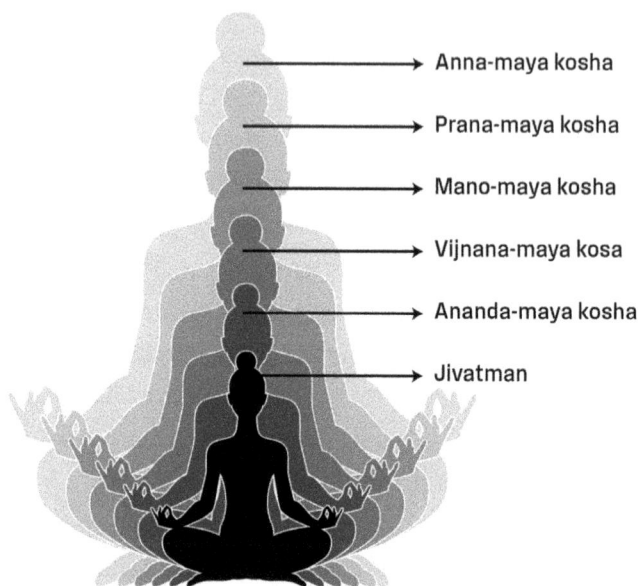

Anna-maya kosha

Prana-maya kosha

Mano-maya kosha

Vijnana-maya kosa

Ananda-maya kosha

Jivatman

HOW DO WE KNOW THE SUBTLE BODY EXISTS?

Your subtle body/energy body is not visible other than in the depiction of koshas shown in figure 3.1, so how can you be sure it exists?

Let's review a basic science lesson. If you dig deep into the hippocampus, the memory storage center forming part of your limbic system located near the amygdala, you may remember learning about the smallest unit of matter known as the atom. Everything that exists is composed of atoms, including humans. Each atom has a nucleus and one or more electrons bound to the nucleus. The nucleus is comprised of protons and neutrons.

- Ninety-nine percent of an atom's mass is found in its nucleus.

- Protons are positively charged.

- Electrons are negatively charged.

- Neutrons have no charge.

Electrons are attracted to the protons by an electromagnetic force, a force that is otherwise known as energy. And here is the kicker: atoms, which comprise all matter, are mostly empty space. That empty space is filled with energy. Because you are comprised of atoms, *you are mostly empty space filled with energy*. Let that sink in.

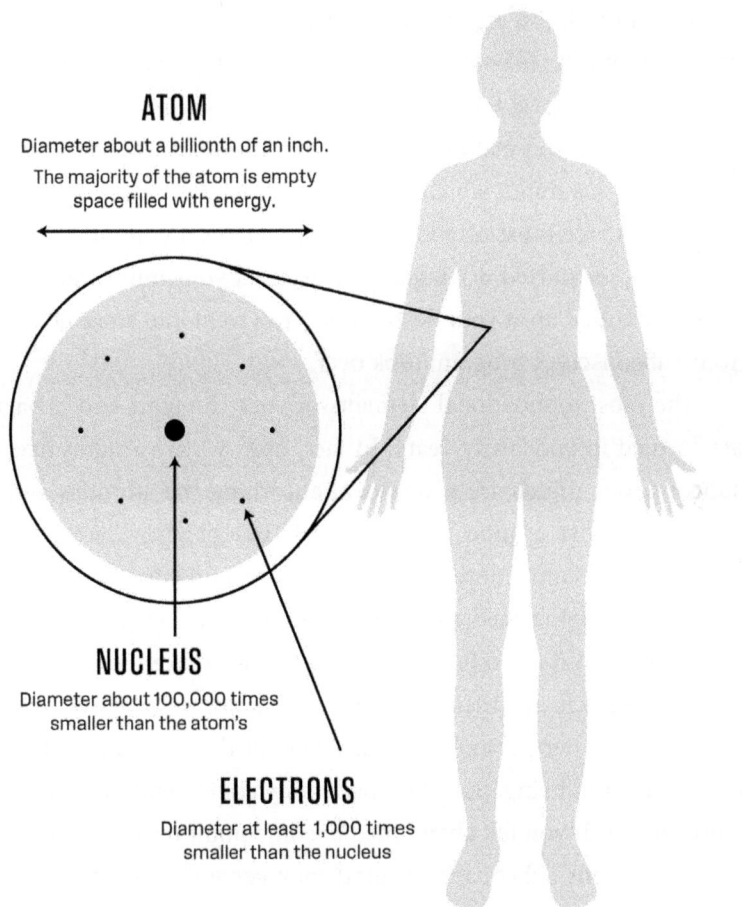

ATOM
Diameter about a billionth of an inch.
The majority of the atom is empty space filled with energy.

NUCLEUS
Diameter about 100,000 times smaller than the atom's

ELECTRONS
Diameter at least 1,000 times smaller than the nucleus

You are mostly your subtle body—your life force energy.

Based on the work of Dr. Bruce Lipton, PhD, author of *The Biology of Belief*,[3] and others such as Gabor Maté,[4] Louise Hay,[5] and Wayne Dyer,[6] we now understand the energetic body, specifically subconscious mind programming, is the primary operator of your being. In collaboration with the amygdala, your subconscious mind continually receives input from the environment and stores all past experiences in a master database. Using that data, it shapes your attitudes and programs your behavior—all without your conscious awareness of the decisions being made. In other words, you don't have to think about your attitudes and behavior. They just *are*.

If you think *you* are in control of your life, think again. Your subconscious mind is in control. According to Dr. Lipton, we operate from a subconscious level 95 percent of the time.[7] Studies show that your subconscious mind makes decisions one-third of a second faster than your conscious mind, which means your subconscious programming will likely drive most of your decisions.[8] Here's a common example: have you ever started driving somewhere, let your mind wander, and suddenly ended up at your destination? You went into autopilot mode. Your subconscious program took over.

The most foundational elements of your thoughts and behaviors are formed in your early years. In fact, until we are around five, our subconscious minds are wide open, absorbing the attitudes and behaviors of those around us, particularly our primary caregivers. By the time we become more consciously aware, our subconscious minds have been programmed with the foundational beliefs that shape our decisions from that point forward—unless we make the effort to understand and change them. Without that awareness, we live our lives based on another person's program. Part of that program may serve our nature and being, but other parts may collide with the essence of who you are. If you felt abandoned at some point during your formative years, your subconscious mind may generate fears of abandonment that impact your sense of safety in later relationships—and you may not be aware of those fears or how they impact you.

Your subconscious mind serves you in other ways too. It includes the ANS, which manages the multitude of body processes occurring in your physical body—from pumping your heart and breathing to controlling body temperature, digesting your food, and more. If you had to think about each bodily function, you would never be able to harmonize your bodily systems.

The subconscious mind contrasts with the conscious mind, which operates in full awareness and allows you to consider and choose your actions. For example, a conscious action might be choosing to go outside and enjoy the sunshine, while a subconscious action might blink against the brilliance of that sunshine.

Think about this: if we operate from a subconscious level 95 percent of the time, *the conscious mind is only responsible for about 5 percent of brain function.* Our lives unfold according to our subconscious programming.

If you are not happy with your life as it is, your subtle body, specifically your subconscious programming, is responsible. If your programming is not in alignment with your prakruti, your birth nature, it will create a state of imbalance, disharmony, and suffering. The resulting inner-brain conflict creates an Ayurvedic imbalance. You gradually become toxic and collect ama at the physical and emotional level, preventing you from connecting with your spiritual self. You get stuck in a state of dosha imbalance known as windy, fiery, or earthy, and you'll wonder how it happened. (Make sure to identify your particular imbalance by taking the stress personality quiz noted in chapter 1.)

The truth is you did not consciously make any of this happen; it happened due to your subconscious program. Your thoughts, your mind, and your physical body are intimately connected. Remember the ancient yogic wisdom defining the koshas or layers of your being we discussed earlier? These layers contain not only the sheath of your physical body, but the energetic layers of breath, mind, intellect, and bliss comprising the subtle or energetic body, which are often missed in Western medicine because of its narrow focus on the physical body.

Just because we refer to these connections as the *subtle* body doesn't mean it is less powerful. In hatha (union of masculine and feminine energies) yoga, breath is used to activate the subtle body. Breath is often used to bridge the gap between the physical outer world and the energetic inner world.

Life force energy, known as prana in Ayurveda and chi in traditional Chinese medicine, sustains us. It provides vitality and vigor. When someone says their energy is depleted, they are referring to a low life force or prana. The subtle body craves a lift in prana, not a cup of coffee, a candy bar, or a Red Bull!

MEET YOUR PRANA

One of the easiest ways to explain how energy or prana is created and utilized in your body is to imagine the action of a wind turbine.

During one of our family's annual hiking trips, we drove from one region of Utah to another and observed many wind turbines along the way.

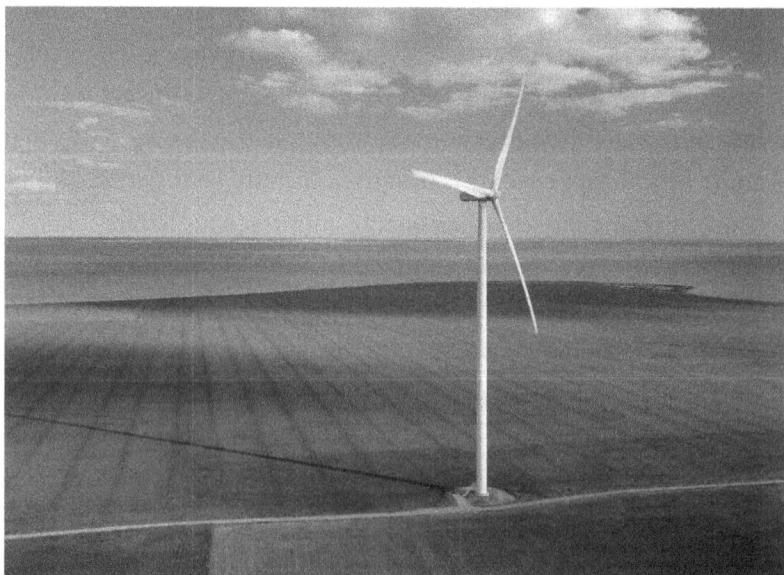

My son, who was about ten years old at the time, wondered what they were for. I told him that wind turbines capture the wind and convert it to electricity. The electric energy could be used to light up a house or warm a space.

When you think of it from an Ayurvedic perspective, the turbines do the following:

They capture air + space + heat elements. These combine to form wind.

Then, it converts wind into electricity, which we cannot see. Thus, electricity converts this energy into light, which not only you can see, it also helps you *to* see.

How ironic.

Without wind, there is no light.

How about that? When your energy is depleted, you do not shine.

Be mindful of the energy you bring into the room. If you want to shine, fill your energy reserve.

If we can accept the idea that electricity exists, despite the fact that we cannot see it, the idea that prana exists should not be surprising. Unfortunately, most people want objective data and the ability to see that something exists—or that it is amiss—in order to accept it as a truth.

MEET YOUR CHAKRA SYSTEM

Your chakra system, a map of 114 points, resides in the subtle body as its emotional/energetic blueprint and energy distribution channel. Seven key chakras are located along the spine. Unaddressed blockages in the chakra system may lead to subtle body disruptions.

Yoga engages mind, breath, and asana practices that cleanses ama, or baggage, and strengthens chakras. Chakras become balanced through these practices, even without focusing on a specific chakra. Similarly, an acupuncturist encourages balance with needles—although they place those needles at specific points. When the chakras are balanced and the meridians or *nadis* open, you will feel a more enhanced flow of energy in your subtle body, and therefore, greater alignment with your mind, body, and spirituality.

BALANCING ENERGY

When you are out of state, you make choices that support your imbalanced energy. That may sound counterintuitive, but have you heard that you resist what you need the most? Or that you crave foods to which you are allergic? When you are disconnected from your subtle body, your sensory body draws you toward the very tendencies that hold you in that state—that is, unless you wake up to the imbalance and proactively make changes to your diet, lifestyle, friends, and so on.

Waking up means becoming conscious of your unconscious program and interrupting its draw toward choices that further imbalance you. When you resonate with low energy, you are drawn to low energy foods, people, and situations. As you shift your inner state, you resonate at a higher vibrational level. This allows you to attract things that are higher in vibration, full of prana and energy, such as more suitable jobs, friends with views and attitudes similar to yours, and freshly grown, nutritious foods over processed foods.

When I struggled with insomnia, I went kickboxing three times per week. I loved it and believed the exercise benefited me. However, my lack of awareness about my stress state made it difficult to assess how helpful the exercise really was. After reading a multitude of books on Ayurveda and discovering I was experiencing a windy-fiery state, I learned that kickboxing was one of the worst things I could do. Kicking and punching only heightened my energy imbalance. Engaging in such aggressive activity told my reptilian brain that I was in danger, so it turned on my sympathetic nervous system—certainly not stress-relieving for my prefrontal cortex!

The Ayurvedic approach suggested I choose activities that turned off those energies and heightened the earthy tendencies that I lacked in my being. Examples of earthy exercises are tai chi and yoga. When I refer to yoga, I am referring to restorative, hatha-type yoga, not hot or intense vinyasa flow yoga. Those aggressive or fast movement oriented yoga practices, just like kickboxing, can further worsen the subtle body state if you are not careful. I started practicing restorative yoga daily, first thing in the morning. I still remember going to the local bookstore, where I spent most of my free time, and buying a yoga DVD filmed amid the beautiful landscape of Jamaica. In the middle of a cold Chicago February, I was transported to a magical place where the lead instructor reminded me, "Yoga is for everyone. You CAN do yoga. The more you practice, the more you will see how you shift . . . achieving bliss and love in your heart."

And, yes, everyone can do yoga. In fact, most of you are doing yoga without even realizing it; it happens whenever you consciously connect your breath and your mind.

The instructor's sweet smile and gentle confidence guided me through the sequence with very different messaging than I received from my kickboxing instructor! The routine felt "cutesy," and the poses didn't seem to accomplish much, yet because I had not slept in three months and was exhausted, I was desperate and willing to try anything. The idea of yoga seemed more appealing than kickboxing anyway. I gave it a go, and I've been hooked ever since.

A CLOSER LOOK AT YOGA

The profound shift practicing yoga stimulates in the subtle body, and eventually the physical body, is beyond words. Ask anyone who has practiced for a while, and they will tell you the same thing. The techniques I learned in yoga allowed me to complete a vigorous four-day trek to Machu Picchu alongside my husband, an Ironman athlete.

Yoga is powerful. Don't let anyone tell you otherwise. You just need to try it yourself to see how it will transform you. Many do not quite understand what yoga does. It opens your subtle body energy and allows it to flow. This nourishes your cells beyond what oxygen and nutrients can do alone. If you are holding onto emotional ama, your physical body will hold it too, blocking this flow of prana or life force. Yoga involves asanas, which open this energy flow.

One goal of improving energy flow is to awaken what is known as kundalini energy. The term *kundalini* comes from the Sanskrit word *kundal*, which means coiled. It is often compared to a coiled snake. The kundalini is considered a powerful form of primal energy or Shakti that sits dormant in your coccyx, at the base of the spine, ready to be awakened. While the snake is often viewed as negative energy, in this case, it provokes us to become more resilient and wiser. If this snake lies coiled and dormant, so will you. You will not awaken to your full potential. You will not be capable of expressing your full, harmonious self. You will continuously feel a void, that something is missing in you or your life. No amount of money, success, or fame can fill that void. I promise you; I have seen the impacts of restricted kundalini time and time again.

Your goal is to unwind, open, and rise, to move from a restricted state to open, awake, and flowing in mind, body, and spirit.

From an Ayurvedic perspective, energy flows through nadis. The human body has 72,000 nadis or channels. Most people spend more time thinking about blood flow and lymphatic flow than energetic flow, however. The main central nadi, known as *sushumna* nadi, is linked to a right-sided nadi known as *pingala* and a left-sided nadi known as *ida*. Practicing breathing techniques, especially in hatha yoga, creates a pause in between breaths, allowing the opening of the pingala and ida energy pathways connecting them to sushumna, the center of the wheel of life.

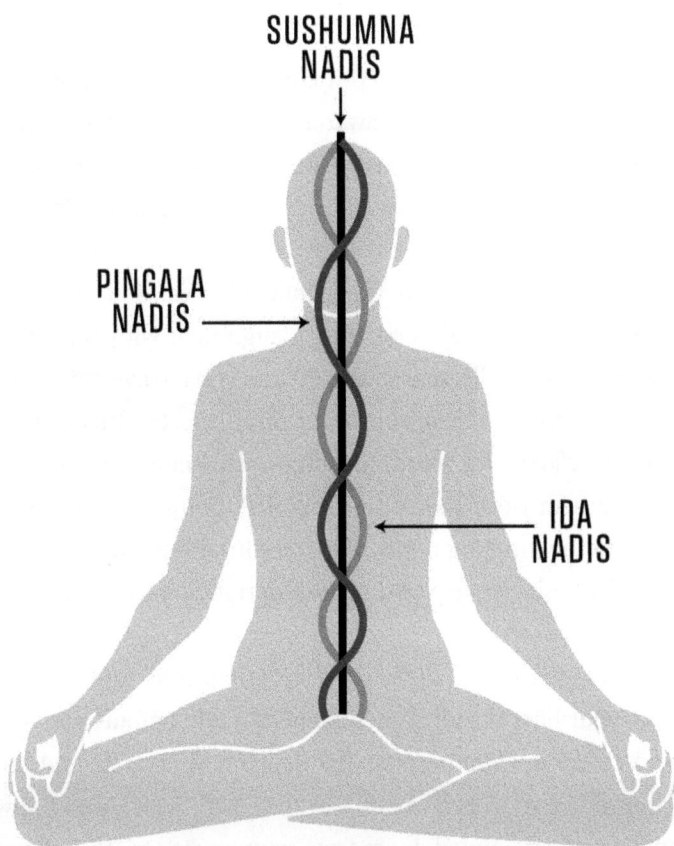

SUSHUMNA
NADIS
↓

PINGALA
NADIS ——————→

IDA
←————— NADIS

You may notice that one nostril is more open than the other, in-dicating a misalignment between the two hemispheres of your brain. To address that imbalance, let's try a simple yoga breathing exercise known as *nadi shodhana*, reverse nostril breathing. Inhale, then close your left nostril and exhale through the right nostril. Then reverse the procedure and notice the difference in the way you breathe. Nadi shodhana balances right and left nadis and creates alignment with the right and left sides of the brain. When practiced daily, it can reduce the conflict between the two hemispheres, lowering the overall struggle within your system, thereby balancing your mind.

THE SUBTLE BODY: YOUR INTUITIVE CENTER

By clearing your nadis of ama, you connect with your subtle energy body. That, in turn, increases awareness of your subconscious program and allows you to more easily connect with your intuitive center, which is linked to your emotional body or your ENS/limbic brain, as previously discussed.

When you clear your ama, the mental, physical, and spiritual conflicts also clear. Your brain operates in alignment with *your* vijnanamaya kosha, your intellectual sheath. When you are overthinking, you are connected to manomaya kosha or mind sheath. This can imbalance the *ajna chakra*, the intuitive center—also known as the third eye. Practicing breath work and connecting with pranamaya kosha allows a quieting of the thinking mind. This frees intuition, thus allowing the vijnanamaya kosha to help you make the right choices and fine-tune your discrimination.

From this place, you are more able to tap into your anandamaya kosha, your bliss sheath. When tapped in, life unfolds with greater flow and creativity. You become less dependent on facts and knowledge from other sources and more in tune with your inner knowing, the innate wisdom handed down from your ancestors. This allows the right brain to open up and be more involved in your being. This creates a balance between the right and left prefrontal cortex and creates coherence. Here, you can operate from a higher level of consciousness, bridging creativity and artistic and innovative thinking with scientific rigor, facts, and knowledge.

Clearing the ama and honoring the subtle body allows you to resonate at a frequency that will enable you to shine bright.

TAKE-HOME POINTS

1. Inner conflict leads to blockages of internal energy flow. This leads to the accumulation of toxins known as ama.

2. Ama can be physical as well as emotional. We sometimes refer to it as "baggage."

3. Ama creates a blockage in the flow of energy (prana or life force) through nadis (energy channels), creating a sense of low energy or lethargy.

4. By creating lower energetic resonance, those inner blocks lead to outer balance. You then attract and are drawn to people, substances, and activity to match that lower energetic level.

5. By removing the ama, a higher energetic resonance is created, thus attracting and being drawn to people, substances, and activity to match.

6. The subtle body is made up of energy in the form of thoughts, emotions, and breath.

7. Your being is composed of koshas or layers. Five layers, moving from the outermost layer of your physical being to the innermost layer of bliss, define who you are through your subtle, energetic body.

8. You have more empty space or more energy than physical structure or matter.

9. To improve your energy and improve your life situation, you must clear your blocks, remove physical and mental ama, and reprogram your subconscious mind.

10. Ninety-five percent of the time, you operate from a subconscious level. It is fundamental to spend time to understand what forms your program, because it guides your behaviors, actions, and thoughts about yourself and the world around you.

SELF-CARE TIME

Practice nadi shodhana, reverse nostril breath. Immerse yourself in this ancient yogic breath technique for two minutes every day. As you practice, imagine clearing your mind and balancing all parts of your brain. You will develop a deeper connection with your breath, and your breath will allow you to connect with your mind. Find the nadi shodhana demonstration and practice video under the chapter 3 list of resources at www.truptigokanimd.com/stressrxbonus.

4

The Stories You Tell Yourself

A bead of sweat rolled down my face on a steamy August day at the Great America theme park in Gurnee, just forty-five minutes north of Chicago. Standing in line, I was unsure if my sweat came from the excessive heat or my impending anxiety about embarking on the new roller coaster, the talk of the town. A long line had gathered. A very long line. My teenage son, Arman, chattered away with excitement, eager to get on board. I, on the other hand—in my early forties—felt a growing sense of unease as the ride spun in circles above our heads, passengers squealing. I did not want to go. My stomach churned as I imagined the force of the ride propelling heads and bodies in multiple directions.

Arman had created a story in his head about the ride. So had I. My story was just as real to me as his was to him. As we waited in line, we felt the same heat from the sun, heard the same screams overhead, and saw the same sights. Yet Arman felt excitement, and I felt fear. What a juxtaposition of emotions!

My thoughts raced, and my heart pounded in terror.

Why had I agreed to join Arman for this risky endeavor?

What was wrong with me?

I thought about walking away, yet how could I leave him in line, alone?

I attempted to soothe myself. *It's just a roller coaster ride after all. Look at the kids and adults exiting the ride with smiles. They all survived. We will too.*

For the next forty-five minutes, as we drew closer to the front of the line, I attempted to calm my mind, and I practiced deep breathing.

Finally, our turn came. We slid into our seats and the attendant latched our lap belts. A few moments later, the car lurched forward. We were off. As we climbed higher and higher, I thought, *My life is over!* Then, we plummeted in mad twists and turns and rose again— prompting an explosion of exhilaration and laughter.

Amazing, and totally unexpected.

When our car stopped at the bottom of the roller coaster, I dismounted with wobbly legs and actually wished we could experience the glorious ride all over again. My boy and I talked about it for days afterward, amused by my initial fear. The story I had told myself beforehand was completely out of alignment with my experience.

Most life experiences are considered neutral. They are neither good nor bad; they just are. As humans who have been programmed with beliefs, thoughts, and attitudes about life and living, we create stories around experiences and events. The roller coaster ride is such an example. One could argue the ride is inherently fear-provoking, yet to an enthusiastic young adult, the ride became one of the most exciting experiences in his life—one creating memories for years to come. For weeks, Arman's friends couldn't stop talking about how enjoyable the ride was and how Arman finally got to experience it.

Why the difference in the significance we placed on the same external event?

It comes down to storytelling.

We all use stories to interpret the world around us. We experience an event that leads to an internal representation of it. This internal representation leads to the story we create. Most of us don't realize how many stories we tell ourselves and are, in fact, completely unaware we are doing it. Every day, each of us overlays actual events or experiences with a story and believe OUR story is the correct one. And it may be.

Yet, what if it is not?

Before we address that question, let's take a closer look at why we tell stories. Storytelling gives meaning to life and expands understanding. Interpretations are shaped by internal programming, and that's where the challenge comes in: your stories represent *your* perception of events and often may not reflect reality.

The reality you create is based on your model of the world (MOW).

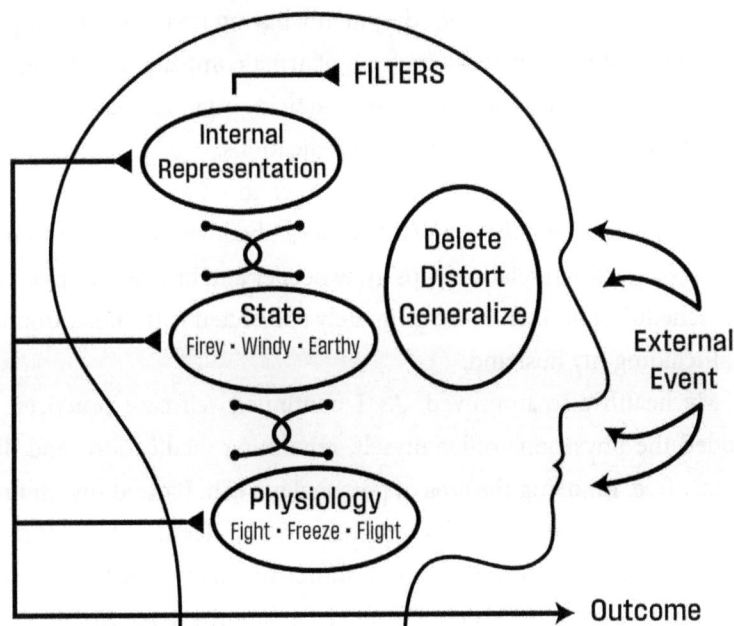

The MOW is a fascinating concept. I spent a few years training in neurolinguistic programming, otherwise known as NLP, and eventually became a master practitioner of NLP. So, what is NLP? Let me explain in the easiest way possible.

NLP = Neuro (Nervous System) + Linguistic (Language)+ Programming (Code or Instructions)

My brilliant trainer, Dr. Matt James, taught that NLP is a model of how your words and thoughts can lead to successful outcomes in your life. Your words do not *describe* the world you live in, but rather, they *determine* the world you live in. This idea is based on how those who succeed actually think, speak, and act, thus allowing success to flow into all areas of life—career, relationships, health, family, personal growth, and spirituality.

Who wouldn't want to learn that model? I was intrigued.

At some level, I knew my life was shifting. I was in my forties, and my career was taking off. My clinic and coaching wait time had expanded despite doing almost no marketing. I was being asked to be a guest on national TV shows, despite my having no media training. I became one of the top speakers for a pharma company despite rarely prescribing the drug. I was, instead, practicing Ayurveda and helping my patients taper their multitude of medications.

Changes showed up beyond my career too. Family connections grew stronger despite the many differences I had with members of my family. My personal relationships grew deeper and broader despite my busy schedule, and I felt more intimately connected with those around me, including my husband.

My health also improved. As I continued self-care practices, I avoided the physician's office myself, remaining medication- and diagnosis-free. Enjoying the area of personal growth, I found myself understanding my purpose in life and how to best live it. I grew deeper spiritually and felt a connection to a source of energy that I had never felt before. Although I couldn't fully articulate the shift, my life was definitely moving in a positive direction.

I believed studying NLP and MOW would expand my understanding and allow me to help others implement the same kinds of changes unfolding in my life.

UNDERSTAND YOUR MOW

Simply put, your MOW is your interpretation of your unique environment. Each one of you has a MOW. Each person's MOW is different from the others. No two individuals have exactly the same MOW because no two individuals share exactly the same experiences and perceptions. You and the person right next to you could share an experience yet have completely different thoughts about and reactions to it.

In his book, *Flow,* Mihaly Csikszentmihalyi says we are all exposed to two million bits of information every second. Due to the high density of data coming in, we can only take in 126 bits per second of the two million.[1]

What do you do with the rest of the information coming in?

You have no choice except to delete, distort, or generalize the information to make it fit into your MOW.

Say you and your friend are walking toward a new bakery that opened the previous week. Your friend notices people gathering around tables inside and enjoying their pastries while a line of people stand outside waiting to be seated. She smells the freshly baked bread and expresses her enthusiasm. She is thinking about how successful the bakery is to have such a nice crowd.

Your friend generalized that a long line + gathering = success.

She may have deleted the stressed faces of the employees and only focused on the smiling faces in the line and the bakery.

Observing the same bakery, you notice the employees running around with anxious expressions. Many more people are standing than sitting. You believe the restaurant is unorganized. They should have waited until they had adequate staffing to open. You didn't notice the smell of bread coming from the bakery.

You generalized that hurried staff + long line = unorganized.

You may have deleted those who were smiling and laughing while standing in line and enjoying their pastries while sitting. Possibly, you even misinterpreted staff facial expressions, assuming their tight features meant they were stressed, when really, they were concentrating deeply.

With so much information to take in, each of you absorbed only what you were able to process by deleting, distorting, and generalizing the incoming information to fit your MOW.

You were both able to give the event meaning and quickly process it. You shared the same walk yet had different experiences.

Which interpretation of the event is correct?

Each of you processed the event to fit your own, unique MOW. It is challenging to say which perspective offers the correct interpretation. In fact, you may both be wrong, or, more likely, the truth is a mixture of both. Where the truth lies isn't easy to pinpoint without fully understanding the experience from all participants' perspectives. You would need to investigate more to find out if the customers were happy or felt unattended. Maybe they were perfectly fine waiting. Maybe they weren't. Maybe the restaurant intentionally scheduled fewer staff to encourage people to slow down and relax or to create a lineup and generate a buzz in the neighborhood. Maybe it didn't. Maybe the staff were stressed, maybe they weren't. Maybe some were feeling one way, and others weren't. It is complex, for sure.

MOW AND BRAIN FUNCTION

Consider this: why did your friend notice the smell of the bread while you didn't?

It's all based on your unique MOW and how it impacts brain function. Your friend's MOW may believe that a busy restaurant is a sign of success based on past observations. Your friend may believe a lineup creates curiosity and excitement about the new business, which only heightened her positive attention to its opening. In that relaxed state, with the five senses fully engaged and ready to receive, your friend's

PFC operated harmoniously with little intervention from the reptilian or limbic brain. Thus, your friend felt at ease with the situation—and that allowed the smell of bread to enter her physiology.

On the other hand, based on your own previous experiences with restaurants and lineups, you may believe customers waiting outside is a sign of poor management. You may have interpreted the staff's serious facial expressions to mean they were stressed. While your friend's PFC remained dominant, your PFC was hijacked by the reptilian and limbic brain. A surge of annoyance and anger prompted your amygdala and subtle body, which stores memories of the past, to shift your physiology into protective mode. In this state, your physiology was tuned into escaping from danger. It told you to keep moving, to avoid stopping to smell (or even taste) the bread!

When you are stressed, your amygdala and your unconscious programming react to perceived danger by constricting your vision. It blocks out the periphery of your vision. You have tunnel vision. You literally *see* less in your world when focusing on area of danger. When your vision is restricted, you see only certain things. Your thoughts are generated based on what you see.

In the face of true danger, I want you to run! Do not stop to experience and observe. Yet, as this story shows, your MOW can prompt you to see danger when danger is not present. We all do this at times, and, to be fair, we do it throughout the day. We are human, loaded with early childhood programming that impacts every aspect of life—from how we respond to a new restaurant to how we respond to an email or text. Unfortunately, as we unquestioningly accept childhood programming, we hardwire inauthentic realities, perpetuating imbalance in the brain.

How often do you add your own story to an event?

How much do you delete, distort, or generalize the truth?

I am sure you have seen MOW at work through social media posts that were intended one way yet interpreted another way by a select few. You may have read the comments and wondered, *what are they thinking?* Perhaps others ask the same question when reading your comments.

Have you watched an episode of *The Real Housewives*? If so, you know what I mean by MOW: the same situation prompts different interpretations, distortions, or meaning-making of the truth.

If danger isn't present, my question to you is this: are you able to create a safer MOW so you can enjoy (and not miss) fabulous bakeries in the future? The answer is yes! You've heard the saying "stop and smell the roses." I would love for you to stop and smell the bread too.

In order to do this correctly—interpret the new bakery—you must create harmony in your system.

HARMONIZE YOUR SYSTEM

In my early years of medical practice, as I began learning about my own programming and MOW, an encounter with a top executive from a global pharmaceutical company showed me how much impact MOW can have. The company was considering hiring me as a speaker to promote a new delivery technology they were bringing to market. The best time for this executive to meet with me was at the end of a full clinic day.

My last patient of the day was a young girl struggling with severe headaches and dizziness, and our consultation ran late. As I exited my office, I noticed the executive reading a migraine journal as he waited. In the past, my MOW would have told me the delay meant I was wasting his time by making him wait. As a result, I would have taken even more of his time by apologizing for running late and offering coffee or tea to assuage my guilt.

But that's not what happened. When I stepped out of my office and saw him reading, I viewed it as an opportunity for him to catch up on new information. I quickly expressed my thanks for his patience and let him know that my patient had needed extra time. I suggested we go outside for a walk to enjoy the beautiful day instead of spending any more time indoors. The suggestion gave me a sense of empowerment, and I noticed his shoulders drop and his smile widen as we stepped outdoors. We had a lovely conversation about family and our hometowns, and eventually, we discussed the new technology.

At the end of our meeting, he told me our interaction was the most meaningful he had experienced in months. He thanked me for taking the time to meet with him and told me he was looking forward to having me on a board of advisors to share the new technology with the world. I became one of the top speakers for the company the following year.

How did this happen? I do not believe I realized it at the time, but after practicing the techniques that I had recommended to my patients and coaching clients, I had begun to shift my own MOW. I began viewing my circumstances differently. Situations that would have triggered my stress personality to emerge in the past no longer did so. That critical inner voice, which would have previously led me to believe I had disappointed or upset someone, now spoke to me in a compassionate and comforting way. Instead of saying, "Oh no, you are running late! You kept him waiting, and now he is bored and has to read to kill time," my inner voice said, "Oh look; he is enjoying a migraine journal."

As the MOW shifts and a compassionate voice rises, there is room for more expansive and beautiful experiences. Defensiveness and protection fall due to a sense of grounding and safety. You stop to smell the roses rather than watching out for potential danger. You see things truly as they are, not as your mind interprets them. The blemished filter is gone.

Early in life, that protective personality, also known as a neurological "part" in NLP, is activated to protect you from danger. The definition of a part based on NLP is: "any state-dependent neural network with enough functional autonomy to run its strategies without control of the rest of the mind." It is a hidden network in your subtle body that you may not even realize is present until you are triggered. Once you begin to reduce your reactive personality and find a more balanced, optimal state, your PFC becomes activated, allowing you to enjoy more of what life offers. Unfortunately, most of you let that personality show up to protect you more than your system requires for safety. More on this later.

Ancient medicine helps you to connect and align with your blissful body as often as possible. This is your true self, the one behind the protective personality. When you are in this state, you feel content, optimistic, safe, hopeful, and energetic. The blissful body is also known as your anandamaya kosha. It resides at your deepest koshic level. Within that layer is your *jivatman*. Your soul. Your truest nature of who you are. Your soul is your North Star. The direction you want to go in life.

Who does not want to be residing at this level as they live in this world?

When you operate from that space, you are more intuitive, creative, flowing, healthy, and energized. You naturally view situations with more clarity and make choices that resonate with your highest self.

Remember, though, there is baggage, a.k.a. ama, which clouds your perception and prevents you from moving inward to that bliss sheath. Your goal is to recognize the cloud and do the work to clear the ama holding you back.

Why do you want to operate from this space? Because you'll have the resources to stay calm no matter what comes your way. Let me share a story.

On a calm Sunday morning, I was busy cleaning out the refrigerator in the kitchen. We had construction workers in the house as the kitchen remodel was underway and progressing smoothly. My husband, an attorney, was in his office, prepping for an important deposition. For the second week in a row, my son went skiing with a dear friend and his mother. As he left, I asked him to confirm that he would wear his helmet. He promised me he would. I also requested he take a few lessons. Although he was naturally athletic, he'd had no formal training on the slopes. He told me he would be fine.

When I looked at my phone, I noticed a missed call from about twenty minutes earlier, around 12:30 p.m. My heart sank. The call was from Mary (pseudonym), the mother of Arman's friend. The previous week, Arman had forgotten his credit card and was kindly treated to lunch. I made sure he had it this time, so why was Mary calling?

My stomach churned. I had a deep knowing that something had happened, so I took a deep breath before listening to her message.

She spoke calmly yet firmly. "Hi Trupti, it's Mary. Please call me back as soon as possible. Thank you."

Her message had no "everything is okay" at the start, which all mothers know to do when there is nothing to worry about. I took another long, deep breath and pressed her number. The phone rang, and she immediately picked up.

"There was an accident," she said.

"Did Arman hurt his head or neck?" I asked. Being a neurologist, the two most concerning areas of impact for me are the head and spine.

"No," Mary gently replied. "He did not hit his head or injure his spine, and he is awake." She continued, calm yet firm. She wanted me to take the situation seriously and make my way up to the ski town, about three hours away.

Arman had skied well all morning. And then, as the universe would have it, he hit a patch of ice and jettisoned into a tree. My son's friend made his way down the hill only to realize his buddy was not behind him, but a few kind young adults saw Arman and called for help.

"The medic team is here and he's stable," Mary reassured me. "It looks like he fractured his femur."

We can get through this, I thought. At least it was not his head or his spine. "All will be well," I whispered to myself.

At this stage, having a few challenging life experiences under my belt, I had learned that my thinking patterns influenced my reality. In medical training, they would always say to check your own pulse before checking your patient's pulse. I finally had tools to keep my pulse in check. I intentionally focused on slow, deep breaths and kept my mind balanced so I could be present.

As I drove up to Wisconsin on my own, doing my best to stay calm, I thought of how challenging it must have been for Mary to wait twenty minutes for me to return her call. I stayed in the moment and did not let my mind wander into potential outcomes.

When I walked into the ER, I knew the injury was severe.

"Oh, YOU are the mother of Arman? He is so brave!" the emergency room front desk nurse said.

It was a compliment, yet I wasn't sure I wanted to hear that before I knew the extent of his injury. I have spent many hours in the emergency room over my years in medical school and residency. This time, it was different. I was not the physician walking in to assess a patient. This time, I was the mother rushing in to see what trauma her son had endured. As I walked into the room where Arman was being evaluated, emotions surged. I held them back. Mary, her son, and the ER doctor were just about to review Arman's films.

As I rushed in, the doctor said, "Here's Mom! Good timing."

Arman looked at me and smiled. It was a strained smile, yet still a smile. A surge of relief swept through me.

His new ski pants were torn off his legs, and he sat on the side of his bed. The film was up on the monitor. Even as a neurologist who had never evaluated leg injuries, I could see the damage. My stomach churned as I took a closer look.

The ER doctor turned to Arman. "Well, you did quite a number on yourself, didn't you?"

The femur was crushed in multiple places, as if he had been in a high-impact motor vehicle accident. I thanked Mary and her son for helping during this time and let them know I would take it from there. I even told them to go and enjoy the slopes. We would be okay.

Emergency surgery was the next step. In the small ski town, there were no available surgeons for this procedure.

"You have two options," the doctor told me. "Have the emergency transport team take him to Children's Hospital of Wisconsin [CHOW]. That's a forty-five-minute drive on a smooth road. Or transport him to

Lurie Children's Hospital in the city of Chicago."

Lurie was a top-rated hospital staffed by many physicians we knew well. I did not know a soul at CHOW, nor did I know about their clinical outcomes. On the other hand, the ride to Chicago would be bumpy and at least two hours. Decisions, decisions.

"I could list off the risks of an unstable fracture, yet since you are a physician, I am not sure you need me to do that," the kind doctor said.

I nodded and asked him not to list the risks. I was, unfortunately, well aware of them. My mind went right to compartment syndrome, where swelling and massive pain in the leg led to the rupture of surrounding vessels and nerves due to the sharp edges of broken bones. I did not allow my mind to explore the depths of what early residency years had forced me to learn. This time, it was my family and I who had to make the decision—and make it quickly.

Many of us have been in a similar place at some point in our lives. We are faced with situations where we have the facts, yet the decision requires something greater. At this moment—like the moment I had ripped up the Prozac prescription—I silenced my racing mind and trusted that inner voice. Instead of weighing pros and cons and using intellectual knowledge, I let intuition guide me.

After a short conversation with my husband, we ended up choosing CHOW in Wisconsin. Arman was taken care of by one of the most seasoned providers in the Orthopedic Department. Turns out, we were in the best hands. The surgery was set for first thing the next morning on Presidents' Day, a holiday, yet the surgeon would come in to take care of my son. We were truly grateful.

Another special touch allowed me to believe we had made the right decision. The floor offered essential oils. I had been recommending essential oils to my patients for years and used them frequently myself. Often, I would have them in my office to help patients breathe through a pain cycle or to calm their nervous system before I administered injections. On the orthopedic floor at CHOW, these oils, if requested, were provided alongside strong opioid medications to help calm the patient's system and reduce pain.

How incredible and surprising to have this offering at a top-notch medical facility!

I spent the entire evening with Arman, helping him practice his breathing when the pain escalated and using the aromas of lavender, peppermint, and vetiver to bring calm, relaxation, and hope to his mind. He woke up every couple of hours as the pain escalated, and then, with the combination of essential oils and opioids, fell swiftly back to sleep while I reminded him all would be well.

Arman's surgery lasted almost an hour longer than predicted, yet I knew he was in highly skilled hands. Afterward, the surgeon told me it had been a difficult surgery, yet he felt confident with the outcome. Arman's growth would not be impacted, and he predicted full ambulation in a matter of two to three months.

Within a week, Arman was released from the hospital. As the universe would have it, just as Arman was to restart school with crutches in hand, the pandemic hit, and a stay-at-home order went into effect. Thus, the remainder of his recovery took place in the comfort of his home. My clinic volume was reduced due to the pandemic, and I was able to attend to Arman to help him fully regain strength.

When I reflect on the experience and ask Arman if he has any negative thoughts or feelings about that time, he repeatedly tells me that he feels nothing but compassion for the team at CHOW. He is grateful that he is now fully ambulatory, and he barely remembers any pain from the event.

I do appreciate that I am asking his conscious mind about the situation, and I don't know what lies at the subconscious level. Yet, for now, I am relieved that the best decision was made at that time with the resources we had. Most importantly, under crisis, I was able to listen to my inner voice for direction. I could only do this because I had managed to shift my reactive personality to a more balanced physiology over the years through my training in Ayurveda and NLP.

Practicing yoga and breath work has strengthened my RAS and

ACC in a way that when danger occurs, even when it is true danger, I can tap into my PFC and call on it to keep me connected to my intuitive self. During times of crisis, whether external or internal, it is essential to remain calm enough to choose the most aligned steps required. With practice and training, everyone can achieve this crystal-clear state of calm.

TAKE-HOME POINTS

1. Most events are neutral. We create a story around the event. Soften *your* story.

2. The story reflects your model of the world (MOW).

3. Due to the high amount of information coming in, you must delete, distort, and generalize information to process what is important to you.

4. Storytelling can lead you to turn on your reptilian and limbic brain, thus hijacking your PFC, the part of your brain that keeps you feeling safe, calm, and joyous.

5. You have the tools to shift your program, clear your ama, and improve your MOW so that it is more in alignment with your true self.

SELF-CARE TIME

Start to notice how you view events and compare them with the views of others—your family, friends, and coworkers—and jot your thoughts down in your journal.

Notice the difference in each individual's MOW.

What do you delete, distort, and/or generalize in your life?

5

The Mistake of Your Intellect

According to Ayurveda, the main reason humans struggle with health, relationships, and careers is due to one principle: *pragyaparadh.*

Pragyaparadh means "mistake of the intellect."

Disharmony in health and life, in general, occurs due to pragyaparadh. If you do not make decisions based on your intellect, life takes you down the wrong path. You choose the wrong partners. You choose foods that imbalance you. You spend time with friends who do not honor you. You move into areas of work that deplete your soul. This leads you to wonder why you don't feel joyful. You will never reach anandamaya kosha—the bliss layer of your being—if this is the direction you go.

The layer aligning with intellect in the subtle body is called vijnanamaya kosha. Intellect goes beyond having the facts. It provides the ability to discriminate between right and wrong based on discernment and wisdom. This kosha is linked to our five senses. We perceive situations via sight, smell, and taste, for example, which then leads to a conclusion. I had utilized these senses when my son was so badly injured, and they allowed me to discern the best next steps for him. Although CHOW was not the obvious choice, I felt a pull to choose it. At the level of my amygdala operating with my subconscious mind, I likely picked up cues from the physician, perhaps even a subtle facial expression indicating he favored CHOW.

I was able to combine the facts and my subtle body's wisdom, allowing my husband and I to make a swift decision that led to a very positive outcome. This force has played out many times in my life and the lives of those around me. When you become connected to the subtle body, you operate from whole-brain intelligence. You make decisions based on your whole self, not on a limited aspect of your personality. Utilizing the physical brain—the subtle energy of the mind, emotions, and intelligence—allows you to reach decisions that lead you in the right direction. In this space, you experience more abundant health, stronger relationships, and more success at home and with your career. You live life with more bliss.

Unfortunately, you will not reach the bliss of anandamaya kosha unless your outer sheaths are healthy and balanced. You must spend time fine-tuning your vijnanamaya kosha (discernment sheath), along with your prana (breath) and manomaya kosha (mental sheath).

Most people focus on the physical body, the annamaya kosha, when they struggle with life. When I asked one woman how she planned on dealing with challenges in her relationships, she responded, "I am going to spend more time at the gym." Unfortunately, lifting weights or doing squats is not the best way to improve relationship challenges. Focus first on brain fitness. Align the mind, the breath, and the intellect to improve relationships, health, and dynamics in the workplace. With an emphasis on subtle body alignment, the physical body strengthens further, and you can reach anandamaya kosha. This approach creates success in all areas of life. It takes effort, but the results are worth it.

DEFINING TRUTH

When it comes to seeking wisdom and aligning with your truth, you may wonder, *what is truth, anyway?* Is truth based on data and science or feeling and intuition?

After researching this topic through my own experiences and training as a yoga teacher, I came to realize that sat (truth) is one of the most important aspects of being a yogini. Speaking, thinking, and behaving truthfully are key to living a yogic lifestyle.

It's always beneficial and often profound to spend some time asking yourself if you are living your truth or the truth of another. Have you been programmed to follow the truth of your parents, your significant other, your boss, your friends, or your pastor? Or are you honoring your truth, which resides within your deepest self?

Behavioral patterns are wired into place during the early years. Programming may even have been absorbed in utero.[1] It is beyond humbling to know that a mother's thoughts and beliefs can be embedded into her developing fetus. If she is stressed and unhappy, she could transmit this to her baby before it has a chance to exit the womb.[2]

Once out in this wild, wild world, the influences of both parents, other caregivers, and society as a whole imprint their programs on a child's being. Children absorb attitudes and behaviors like a sponge and only begin to wake up to them in their teens. They either agree with their programming or disagree with it. That's when the internal battle and teenage rebellion begins.

Or they could react like I did.

I excelled at being a pleaser. I squashed my emotions deep. You see, I, like many others, did not have a safe environment to discuss feelings. At that time, emotional expression and vulnerability were generally believed to be signs of weakness, not strength. Thus, families—especially the immigrant ones we spent time with—learned to push through discomfort and stayed outward-focused. They did this by accommodating other people and performing to meet their expectations—and putting on a smile while they did it.

When trauma occurred in a family, which it often did, no one discussed it. Ignoring trauma and continuing to live as though it weren't happening felt surreal. I did not gain access to my own voice until much later in life. After many years of self-work through yoga, meditation, coaching, reading personal growth books, and attending presentations, I finally began to speak my truth. I finally stood up for the real me, not the personality I had once thought protected me. It took me years to discover my truth, who I am, and why I am here on this earth—and I'm still working on it. But once I began waking up, I began feeling true bliss for the first time in my life.

We spend years sacrificing a connection to ourselves and instead forcing a connection with others through perfecting, pleasing, and caretaking. We squeeze ourselves into the mold of a person others want us to be versus simply being ourselves. In order to stop that cycle, we must awaken to who we really are.

> *"To be yourself in a world that is constantly trying to make you something else is the greatest accomplishment."*
> *—Ralph Waldo Emerson*

Fortunately, we can change our programming at any age.

What is truth? It is more than just facts. It is a blend of the knowledge obtained from books or mentors and our inner knowing or wisdom. With knowledge, we accumulate facts based on proven ideas or concepts. We choose to agree or disagree with knowledge according to the data we decide to read and what has been studied. Wisdom, however, is not based on facts. It is based upon our connection to the subtle body, its ability to receive information from source, from the universe.

Wisdom is tied to intuition. Ancient sages of India received wisdom from the universe after spending hours in deep meditation and connecting with their truth. Ayurvedic sages observed that individuals fell into one of three doshic constitutions: vata, pitta, or kapha. This was cognized by observing and receiving wisdom from source. We can all tap into this innate wisdom, and we do not need to meditate hours per day to accomplish this.

Wisdom allows creativity and innovation. Wisdom allows growth and expansion beyond what has already been proven and studied. It allows individuals to fully connect with their truth and shows them how to live and align with their purpose. Alignment with purpose provides the ultimate freedom, confidence, and bliss.

"The intuitive mind is a sacred gift, and the rational mind is a faithful servant. We have created a society that honors the servant and has forgotten the gift."
—*Albert Einstein*

Friends, let us not forget our sacred gift.

YOUR STORIES, TRIGGERS, AND TRAUMA

Unfortunately for many, the inner voice of the soul is not heard. Too many competing voices vigilantly protect against perceived danger and drown out the calm and harmonious inner voice.

The best way to access your voice is to start asking what triggers (activates) you. What stirs your mind and keeps you stuck in a certain thought pattern for days? Those triggers are indicators. They allow you to reflect on which parts of yourself need repair. It is easy to get caught up in the stories of your MOW and focus on triggering events. You point your finger at the event or individual instead of asking how you allow yourself to be triggered.

It is human. Most people do it. The key to stopping is to see the pattern and break it. Only then can you be free from the pattern that is leading to an imbalance in your mind and, eventually, your body.

WHAT IS A TRIGGER?

I was having coffee with a dear friend and discussing a relative whom she had recently seen. "Every time I spend time with him, he pushes my buttons," she said. It seemed that each time this relative approached her, my friend noticed her energy shift. Her shoulders tightened and her breath shortened as she expected to be criticized or judged.

We all know what being triggered means. At some point, each of us has likely felt triggered by external situations, events, or individuals that push our buttons and bring up uncomfortable emotions. Some people feel constantly triggered. For others, it's an occasional experience.

What exactly is a trigger?

A trigger is a sensory experience that activates a deep subconscious part of your neurology. It could be a voice, a sound, a sight, a feeling, a taste, or even a smell, and it's based on what your amygdala and limbic system are holding onto from past circumstances. Your reaction to this seemingly innocent sensory experience—whether fear, anxiety, anger, or depression—may be out of proportion. Depending on the severity of the trigger, it may take you longer than expected to return to your baseline.

One of the biggest reasons you remain in conflict, fighting an internal battle, is because you carry triggerable neurological parts, the subconscious programs created by stressful or traumatic experiences. Many of these experiences are beyond memory. You may have been abandoned on the playground when you were five, for example, and now you fear your friends will leave you. I will never forget rushing home from my office on a cold February day. I was running late with a patient, and my daughter's bus was to drop her home by noon. She was in kindergarten and in a half-day program. I frantically called a couple of neighbors, yet no one answered. As I pulled closer to my home, I saw my sweet five-year-old girl sitting on the front step in her pink, fluffy coat. She looked up at me with tears in her eyes as I pulled into the driveway. For a few weeks after this incident, she would cling a little tighter when I dropped her off. I reassured her that she would be fine and that I would certainly be home when she finished school. I would wait outside when the bus pulled up, and she slowly let her fear of abandonment dissipate. These theories are further elaborations of the subconscious mind work of Sigmund Freud and Carl Jung.

Certain individuals or situations may activate a large number of people in the same way. You may agree with your friends, family, or co-workers that a particular individual is toxic and difficult to be around. In this scenario, ask yourself questions to determine why you are reacting. *Why is this individual or that situation occurring in my life? What can I learn from this? How can I improve myself so this external activator can be less triggering?* This may seem hard to do, yet this is how to evolve past blocks and create more peace within us and our lives.

We all carry positive and negative memories that impact future events. I remember eating the most delicious paella with a savory aioli sauce in Valencia. My medical school friends and I sipped on sangrias as a breeze came in through an open window in the beautiful Spanish restaurant on the coast. When I returned to the states and had paella there, I immediately remembered the bliss of that moment, and the memory brought me back into the state of that moment.

Now imagine the opposite scenario.

My husband loves making cocktails. For some of our friends, adding tequila makes them grimace. They want nothing to do with it. It's too close to experiences of the late-night tequila drinking in college. Most likely, those experiences were linked to physical and emotional discomforts that became deeply lodged in the memory banks of the limbic brain. They are triggered by the thought, smell, or sight of tequila. Even just talking about the experience can be triggering.

Triggers activate a part of our neurology. There is always an emotion tied to the part, and it is stored in the subconscious mind and physiology.

On another occasion, I told a group of friends about a time when a colleague, who was about ten years my senior, told me he loved my new hairstyle. One friend felt strongly that this statement was disrespectful and chauvinistic. I told her that I was flattered and had thanked him! I hadn't heard any disrespect in his manner or tone. I let him know that

I had finally found a stylist who knew how to do my hair, and I was grateful he noticed. For my girlfriend, his behavior was triggering; for me, not at all. There was no right or wrong in this situation: simply, she was triggered, and I wasn't.

We each have different scenarios that push our buttons because we each carry a different MOW. We interpret signals and situations based on this model. My friend may have had an early life experience where she felt belittled by an older man, possibly a father figure. Thus, her neurological part was defined and became a triggerable area for her. More on this later.

Remember: triggers activate our parts. These parts carry memories from the past tied to an emotion. With the trigger, you begin to generate stories based on how triggered you get, whether they are stories about others or stories about the world.

In the doctor's office, we ask patients what triggers their migraines, anxiety, or digestive issues. We encourage them to reflect on various external factors that allow their brains and bodies to become more activated. When providers do this, they place the locus of control on something external. Doing so trains patients to respond with statements such as, "My migraine came on because it was raining," "My hormone cycles always lead to a migraine," or "My boss was being difficult, and that triggered my pain."

For years, I asked my patients about their triggers and helped them connect to their pain by becoming aware of their activators. At some level, this is appropriate. It provides awareness of the scenarios that allow feelings of imbalance. However, it doesn't provide the full story. Let's take alcohol, for example. If you have had a long day at work on the first day of your menstrual cycle (if you cycle), staying out late for cocktails with friends after work may not be in your best interest. Alcohol, in that scenario, may trigger a sleepless night or a headache the following day. Contrast that with having an after-dinner glass of wine while relaxing with your significant other on your patio. In that scenario, alcohol may relax you and allow you to sleep deeply, feeling refreshed and pain-free in the morning.

Yet, if you consume alcohol often in scenarios similar to the first—when it has a negative impact on you—your MOW may say that alcohol triggers you and you should stay away from it.

Do you see how a story gets created that may not serve you?

Thus, focusing on external triggers or activators may lead you down a path where you start to blame the world for your problems instead of looking more closely at yourself.

I think of this quote by the brilliant Sufi philosopher Rumi: "Yesterday, I was clever, so I wanted to change the world. Today, I am wise, so I am changing myself."

Instead of believing your headaches or any other symptoms were triggered by the rain, consider how you were more vulnerable to symptoms due to your lack of sleep and skipping meals. This situation lowered your pain threshold and allowed the weather shift to manifest a migraine—like the proverbial straw that broke the camel's back. It is easier to point fingers at someone or something—especially something like the weather, which can't argue back!

This may be hard to hear. I have been there. When I suffered from insomnia, I wanted nothing more than to blame my sleep on the lighting in the room, my low magnesium levels, and the stress of medical school. Because I blamed external circumstances, I came close to quitting medical school. Thankfully, I did not. Ayurveda taught me to pause and look within for an answer instead of searching for the answer "out there." It taught me to work on myself versus running away from the trigger. If I had run away from the trigger, I would have never become a medical doctor, and I wouldn't be writing this book.

I encourage you to start concentrating on your internal state. Explore your experiences and your MOW to discover how much imbalance you may be carrying versus trying to find the answer externally. Focus on strengthening your internal system to become less triggerable rather than fighting the uphill battle of extinguishing triggers. I promise you, you will have greater success. I have seen it time and time again.

When triggers are linked to particular scenarios or individuals, you may want to ask what you have to learn from that situation or person.

Is that individual or situation appearing in your life to teach you something?

Or to evolve you in some way?

You may be telling yourself if the world were better, you would be better. For example, if you didn't have to work with that annoying person at the office, or if your husband were more helpful around the house, you wouldn't have stress, anxiety, pain . . . you fill in the blank. Instead of focusing on the world, try taking a look inward and ask yourself how you are allowing yourself to be triggered by the world around you. Ask how you can change yourself rather than trying to change the world.

I know this is true because this is my story.

CONFRONTING THE VICTIM

In my early years, I wasted so much energy complaining about the inadequacies of others and how they wouldn't contribute or step up. As a recovering perfectionist, I felt most of the people I worked with were not driven enough or passionate enough for life, work, and relationships. Thus, I always felt the urge to complain about their lack of commitment. I saw fault readily and believed everyone else should be "better."

At some level, dissatisfaction with the status quo is good. It allows us to level-up and improve the current situation. As chief resident in neurology, for example, frustration motivated me to encourage my fellow residents to be more present for their patients, respond to pages faster when emergencies arose, and record more diligent notes.

We can elevate standard care and outcomes in all areas of life in response to dissatisfaction. Yet, expecting outcomes that are beyond what we can handle creates the perfect setup for stress, doesn't it? There is a fine balance between complaining, venting, and storytelling versus issuing a challenge to feel motivated or resourceful.

Herein lies the key.

Simply complaining and venting about someone or something not being good enough only hardwires your circuitry for believing the world is "not good enough" for you. Indulging that story gives it a stronger pull for you and initiates what I call the victim mindset or personality. You may even recruit others who share similar perspectives, thereby further hardwiring this belief into your circuitry.

This strengthens the neurological part. It is this vulnerable, triggerable area that gives you internal conflict. In the discipline of NLP, we were trained to find parts hidden in the subconscious psyche. There may be one part monitoring safety that prevents you from stepping too far out of your comfort zone. As a result, you choose to live in the same house, go to the same restaurants, and keep the same job— even though you are itching for change because those things are safe and comfortable. Another part does not want you to feel abandoned, so you limit your friend circle to people whose support you can rely upon 100 percent of the time—even relationships that may be toxic. You may feel unsafe and fear abandonment, thus staying with the same abusive partner for a false sense of security and companionship, even though it is traumatic. I have clients who eat certain foods or drink certain beverages regularly for a sense of security and comfort, even though those choices are unhealthy for them.

Certain neurological parts may have been created to keep you cautious about romantic relationships, leading to trust issues with new partners. Certain parts may keep you taking the same medication for years, even if you aren't sure it still works, as you feel a sense of safety by taking it. The goal is to loosen the charge and intensity of that part while loosening the pull or grip these parts have on your well-being. In that way, you can approach new challenges without feeling unsafe.

You can bring people into your life without fearing abandonment. You can move into relationships with more trust. You can confidently taper your medications when you are ready.

One way of approaching this conflict is by clearing the part with some hypnotic NLP parts techniques. Another approach, which took me many years to learn and a few coaches to reinforce, is to step into the unease and ask yourself what can be done about it. It is important to observe your behavior and stop playing the victim card. Instead of sharing your discontent and stories with friends and family or the cashier at the supermarket, explore how you can improve the situation and your thoughts about it to relieve your disease. The victim personality brings out an unattractive and unproductive side of your nature, and it creates stories about your experience.

Stories protect you from emotional pain; however, the more you tell yourself a particular story, the longer you remain stuck in it. Your body holds your emotional pain physically. The energy of suppressed emotions moves into various body parts, and your energy body, which is quite intelligent, uses physical pain to warn you that you are out of alignment and in danger.

Do you have neck pain and tightness or lack of mobility when turning your head from side to side? This is your energy body's warning that vata energy (air and space elements) are in excess. If you don't take care of the situation, the excess may move into your brain and mind, creating worse problems. So, remember this: your energy body does all it can to protect you. Your subtle body sends a gentle message through pain or tightness, nudging you to move away from danger before problems escalate.

After taking care of countless individuals struggling with symptoms from anxiety to cognitive challenges to digestive imbalances, I have a few words of advice: do not surrender to your world. Do not tell yourself *this is just how it is*. Do not accept a trigger and believe that these activators are present to create disharmony and discontent. This is simply not true. In fact, it is quite the opposite. These triggers alert you to your part, which needs some attention and balancing. The more you work on yourself, the better your life and your world will be. I have seen magic happen with my patients. The more balanced and harmonious you become, the more balanced and harmonious your world will be. It just is.

This is the message of the ancient wisdom book, the Bhagavad Gita, and it is the same message shared by spiritual teachers from many unique backgrounds. It's all about understanding what your conflict is and resolving it. It may be one main conflict, or, oftentimes, many little conflicts or *micro-stressors*. They keep your brain in a heightened state, ready to react. It takes time to uncover the conflicts, yet it's worth the effort.

Socrates, one of the greatest philosophers of all time, once said, "An unexamined life is not worth living."

If you do not take the time to examine yourself, you will never truly be healthy, happy, or prosperous. You may end up spending thousands of dollars on medical bills and prescriptions, changing jobs and partners, raising imbalanced kids, and perpetuating patterns of disconnect.

I hope this book allows you permission to break these patterns, soften the parts, and reduce the charge of your triggers. This is the key to resolving inner conflict. It begins with recognizing your stories and allowing yourself to shift your MOW to create harmony.

TAKE-HOME POINTS

1. Pragyaparadh, a mistake of the intellect, is believed to be the cause of disease based on Ayurveda.

2. Truth is the combination of knowledge and wisdom.

3. Situations that trigger you allow you to reflect on which parts of you need repair.

4. The neurological parts are hardwired into your subconscious mind based on past events and trauma.

5. Stories can hardwire the part; be careful with storytelling and blaming the trigger as the cause of your ailments.

6. Your goal is to recognize the triggerable part and soften it by shifting your reaction to the trigger, rather than attempting to remove the trigger altogether, as that is impossible to do.

SELF-CARE TIME

As you practice the following self-care exercise, pay attention to how you feel and what you are thinking. If it feels too difficult, move to the sections allowing you to focus on your breath and body versus going directly into your thoughts and emotional patterns.

Note: You may also consider working with a coach or therapist to help you work through these areas.

Allow yourself to connect to your physical body and begin to move into the subtle body. The easiest way to do this is with your breath.

Start with practicing reverse nostril breathing.*

After doing this breathing exercise, grab a journal and identify what triggers you:

- Which events, people, or situations trigger an emotional response?

- How many triggers do you have?

- Write down any situations, scenarios, and people challenging you now.

- How do you respond to being triggered? List any physical,

---

* See the link to a video illustrating reverse nostril breathing at www.trupti-gokanimd.com/stressrxbonus.

mental, and emotional responses. How do you feel physically, mentally (with your thoughts), and emotionally (with your feelings) about the situation?

- How often are you exposed to these triggers?

Remember that if a charge exists, that is a good thing. It means you know where to focus your clearing efforts. When you clear this baggage, you can feel energized and empowered. You will release the energy spent suppressing the part and use that energy for more creative endeavors.

Remember Arjuna in the Bhagavad Gita—the story shared in chapter 2? Just as he chose to fight for what was right rather than surrender to the conflict, so can you.

6

Trauma: Who Doesn't Have It?

Trauma is a pervasive and universal problem. My life began in survival mode, yet it did not occur to me until years later how the circumstances of my birth would affect me for years to come. I had no idea the story I carried provoked such disharmony in my being—until the day I decided to share it.

I sat with a friend, a fellow resident from Nigeria, in the noisy VA hospital cafeteria with our typical lunch of steak fries and ketchup paired with a beet salad. People buzzed around us. After an interesting few hours caring for psychiatric patients, we sat quietly in the cafeteria, contemplating the morning. Most of our patients were admitted with a history of severe post-traumatic stress disorder (PTSD). It led to delusions and psychosis, often sprinkled with manic features, and it caused distress in their home environment. It was so disheartening to witness their struggles on a daily basis that we rarely spoke about our personal challenges. The patients needed our full attention.

The kind-hearted resident looked up from his meal and asked, "Where were you born?"

I smiled. "Africa," I replied, feeling a sudden connection to my Nigerian friend.

He shared a quizzical look. "Africa? Wait, aren't you from India?"

I told him that my parents and grandparents were born in Africa. I was born in Kampala, Uganda, where my father worked as a physician with a busy medical practice. He enjoyed caring for the community while my mother taught home economics. They had three servants, one of whom took care of me and my older sister. One tended to the house and garden, and another servant prepared all our meals. Mom would pick sweet, ripened mangoes on her way to school as she would teach her classes outdoors.

Until that moment, the conversation was light and fluid. However, as I began to describe Idi Amin, the dictator who led a military coup and seized power a few months before my birth in 1971, I teared up. He had given my family three months to leave the country simply because we are South Asian. The Ugandan Asian exodus took place because Idi Amin believed South Asians threatened local Ugandans by taking away employment and business opportunities and hurting their ability to succeed. It was ethnic cleansing, which Amin modeled after Hitler's regime.

When my father tried to obtain a travel visa for me as a newborn, so we could leave the country, he was told that could not be done. After a mild altercation, he was thrown in jail.

Usually, the government killed anyone they imprisoned.

Tears streamed down my face. My fellow resident shook his head and teared up too.

Dad bribed the jail guard with keys to our car and was eventually released. He was fortunate; atrocities were committed against anyone during that time who resisted the new regime. Idi Amin had even killed his wife. He put her mutilated body on display for his son to view, making it clear that any dissent from his coup was a reason to be killed.

Tears continued to flow as I talked about that time. I stopped periodically to catch my breath and still my trembling voice.

My friend grabbed my hand. "It's okay," he said, trying to console me.

With no sense of where to go or any means to exit, my family suddenly had to pack up and leave within ninety days. Mom risked her life sneaking me through the customs line, as they had not found a way to gather the travel documents I needed to fly.

Somehow, before that moment in the cafeteria, I had never allowed myself to share so much detail about my early life. This kind resident gently pursued more information, showing compassion and empathy as I spoke my story out loud.

As I continued to share, something overcame me, and I couldn't talk. I silenced myself—and then began crying uncontrollably. I mean, full-on sobbing right there in the cafeteria! I had no idea what had come over me, and I had no way of stopping it either. I had never experienced such a dramatic wave of sorrow, especially in a public place.

Mind you, I was only a *few months old* when Mom smuggled me out. I had no conscious recollection of the event, yet overwhelming emotions traveled through me as though I were vividly recalling every moment of our escape. I was beyond surprised by my reaction, but I felt a sense of relief when I finished sharing.

Why did this storytelling about an event I believed had no impact on me lead me to such an outpouring of emotion?

Perhaps some part of me, separate from my conscious awareness, compartmentalized the experience and held onto a full memory of this stressful period of my life.

Until I shared that story with my fellow intern, I had been unaware I carried any memories of the event. After all, I was only a few months old at the time. It had been years since my family discussed the events, and even then, my parents only shared a high-level perspective of the experience. Never had it generated the emotions I felt in the cafeteria. Exposure to a few books on Idi Amin in middle school while researching a paper had no impact either. I treated the assignment as though I were an observer, not an active participant.

So, why was I suddenly getting so emotional about the story while sharing it with my friend?

The resident grabbed my hand. "I am so very sorry that you and your family went through this. I can't even imagine the impact this has had on all of you."

I eventually settled myself down, and we finished our lunch.

It took me years to understand how trauma lodges itself in neurology. How it innocently hides in subconscious programming. It can lurk under the surface and allow us to believe we are past it, but the subtle body remembers. It holds onto emotions and perceptions far longer and more deeply than we realize at the conscious level. It retains feelings and memories in a way that our conscious mind may never recall. That is the truth.

TRAUMA—IT'S PERVASIVE

According to the National Council for Mental Wellbeing, 70 percent of adults in the United States have experienced some type of trauma.[1] Episodes of trauma lead to the development of neurological parts— different areas in the brain involved with these memories, feelings, and reactions that may not be consciously remembered. Eventually, these parts become triggers for you.

I first learned about trauma, in the context of PTSD, during my psychiatry training. In my mind, trauma was limited to those who experienced abuse, were at war, raped, or exposed to other forms of violence. I was limited in my perspective of who could experience trauma. To me, if it wasn't a significant event, it wasn't trauma. I also believed one had to have firsthand experience and conscious recollection of trauma to have been traumatized.

That is far from the truth.

As I have worked with patients over the years, my definition of trauma expanded. Let's take a look at what trauma means in relationship to stress.

STRESS AND TRAUMA

Dr. Hans Selye, a Hungarian endocrinologist, studied the impact of stress on biological systems. Often referred to as the father of stress, he offers a simple yet meaningful definition of stress as a situation that occurs when the demands placed on an organism exceed what it can manage.

When an organism encounters stress, it adapts by releasing hormones, neurotransmitters, and cortisol intended to help it recover from the stressful event and move back into harmony.

Now, let's relate that to the idea of trauma. I offer a definition drawn from the brilliant observations of Dr. Selye: trauma occurs when the demand placed on an organism (individual) is more than the organism can handle, leading to a near persistent state of imbalance mentally, physically, and emotionally.

In other words, internalized trauma occurs when exposure to something traumatic triggers an ongoing state of imbalance with no return to the baseline balance or homeostasis once the event has ended. Contrast this with the definition of stress, where the body moves back into homeostasis after a demand is placed on its system.

Keep in mind that the demand is not always external. In fact, most of the time, it is internal. Negative thoughts, for example, reflect an inner demand.

With state imbalance, you enter into a windy, fiery, or earthy state to protect yourself from perceived danger. The nervous system reacts by immobilizing, attacking, or moving you away from danger. Another way of thinking about these reactions is freeze, fight, or flight. All living things move into these states to hide, defend, or escape from threats. The organism freezes to become small. It hides to avoid being seen. When an organism fights, it chooses to engage in outwardly aggressive behaviors to ward off the danger. In either of these states, escape is not possible. The organism takes flight when it moves away and withdraws from the perceived danger. Ghosting someone is a form of flight and escape. Watching Netflix to "numb out" is an escape, as is using cannabis or alcohol to temporarily disengage from life's challenges.

Watching Netflix or occasionally enjoying wine or cannabis is not the problem. The problem arises when someone partakes in these activities to disengage from perceived stressors in life, especially when repetitively resorting to these measures as an escape.

Dissociation from self is another method used to escape danger. This is done by taking on an outward personality that strives for perfection, caretaking, people-pleasing, or even humor such as sarcasm. These personalities or traits hold one in a state to avoid processing difficult emotions or feelings that lead to discomfort or pain. Unfortunately, emotions only become further stuck in the subtle body, which leads to physical disease development if not cleared.

A recent study published in 2021 revealed that perfectionistic self-presentation, defined as "the drive to appear to others as perfect," is linked to pediatric pain syndromes.[2] This is just one of many articles published on this topic. To date, countless studies evaluate these various personality types and disease manifestations.

I encourage you to look into the publications of Dr. Gabor Maté, MD, one of the leading experts on this topic. His book, *When the Body Says No*, is one of the most influential explorations I have ever read about the interaction between our stress response system, emotions, and disease presentation.[3]

The Traumatized Personality

Now you understand how trauma can become lodged in the subtle body and make you more prone to being triggered. This leads to the development of a protective personality. As I explained before, triggers can be internal and external. Weather change is an external trigger for those who are sensitive to it. Internal triggers involve shifts in your bodily functions, such as hormone excretion or digestion, for example. Keep in mind that your five senses process the triggers. What you see, taste, feel, smell, and hear externally or internally alerts you to potential danger. Your subconscious neurological pattern may have programmed certain sensory memories that you interpret as being dangerous to your being.

ADRENAL STRESS
ACUTE STRESS EVENT

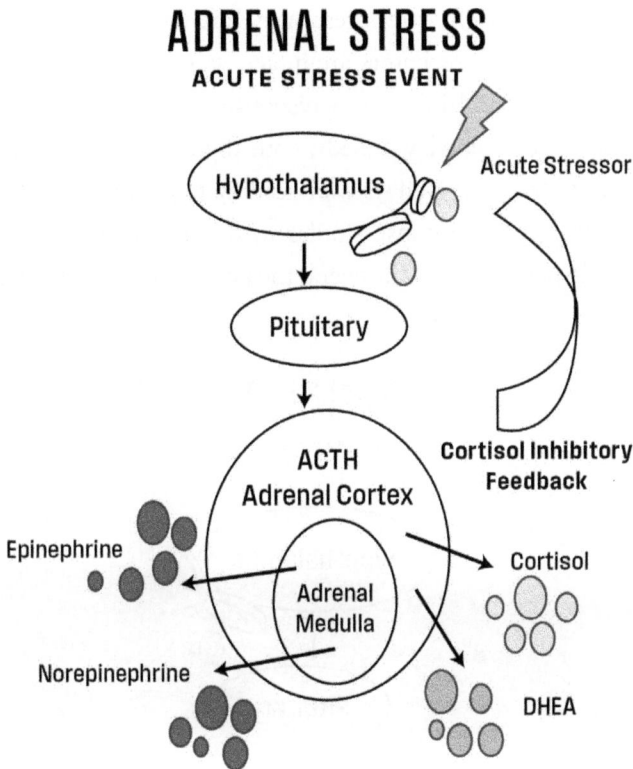

As you can see from the image above, after encountering an acute perceived stressor, the hypothalamus (which I call the divine internal mother) activates the pituitary gland. The pituitary is the master of all hormones. It releases adrenocorticotropic hormone (ACTH), which then turns on the adrenal glands. When a physiological stress response occurs, norepinephrine is released by the adrenal medulla yet disappears within an hour or so after the stressor subsides. Cortisol, released from the adrenal cortex, the stress hormone that mimics a steroid similar to prescription prednisone, is released and may not disappear for forty-eight hours.

A cortisol inhibitory feedback loop, in which the cortisol released by your body signals the brain to prevent further release of the stress hormone, generally *dampens the cortisol release.* Your system basically tells you to turn off the stress response, hoping the stressor is over. If your hypothalamic receptors are intact, your body is responsive to that signal and turns off the stress response. Even though the adrenal hormones reduce relatively quickly, your digestive system often stays inflamed after the perceived stressor, leading to gut inflammation.[4]

Stress triggers a response similar to the one above. If the stress doesn't come from a traumatic event, the body moves swiftly back into homeostasis or a steady state.

ADRENAL STRESS
HOMEOSTASIS

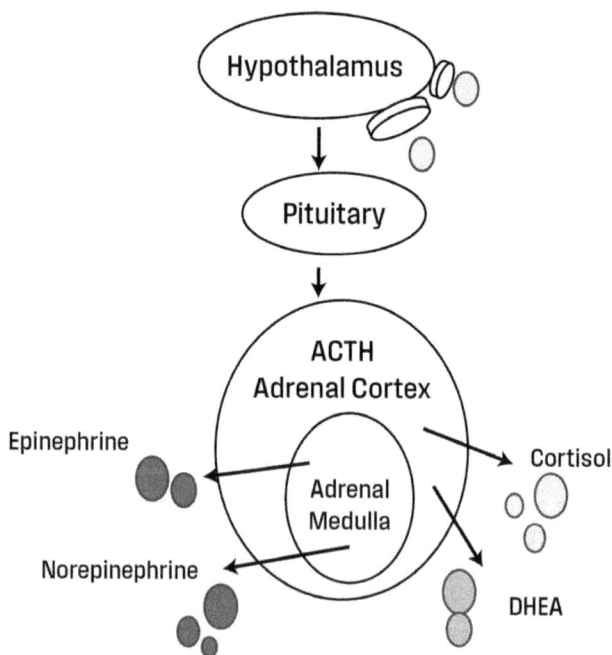

In a traumatic situation, stress is experienced, yet the system moves out of state. When the trauma passes, the body shifts into an imbalanced physiology and carries the burden of the trauma within the energetic (subtle) and physical body. This leads to the development of the persistent fiery, windy, and/or earthy state imbalance.

A recent Gallup poll showed that eight out of ten Americans said that they were affected by stress. Eight out of ten Americans—and that was in 2017, before the COVID-19 pandemic.[5] After the pandemic, the mental health crisis has worsened. The average lifespan dropped by two years.

In addition, 40 percent of job turnover is due to stress.[6] Workplace stress accounts for up to $190 billion in health care costs.[7] Even if you believe you were lucky enough to avoid trauma in the past, living through the pandemic, along with its aftermath, has likely left a traumatic imprint on your subtle body that may not manifest for years to come.

The world is stressed and traumatized. This is just a fact. Unfortunately, these conditions are gaining momentum not just with adults but also our elderly and children as well.

Intergenerational Trauma

We face not only the trauma experienced in our own lifetimes but also the potential trauma passed down into your neurology from past generations. This is known as intergenerational trauma.

Think about it. Why did I start sobbing while telling the story of my parents' trauma?

It was because I carried the burden of my mother's trauma. In utero, the developing fetus picks up on the emotions and energy of the mother. Neuroimaging studies even reveal potential changes in the amygdala and hippocampus size in the offspring of mothers who have experienced trauma.[8]

My sudden explosion of tears resulted from holding an unrecognized trauma for years. The kind and receptive psychiatry colleague, with his compassion and open-heartedness, created a safe space that allowed me to feel comfortable enough to discuss the traumatic experience. This gave me the ability to release the sadness that my energetic body had clung to. It didn't make sense at the time, yet now it is clear.

Even though someone may not consciously believe they are carrying trauma, the subconscious mind will let them know at times like these.

After my experience in the hospital cafeteria, I was able to share this story a few more times with dear friends and family. It took years to do this without a powerful emotional response, yet now, no crying or emotions of any sort emerge when talk about it. I have been able to clear the unprocessed energy from my physiology, my subtle body.

If emotions surge while you tell a certain story, or if you won't allow yourself to talk about it, there is a charge to the story. The charge is baggage that needs release from your physiology.

That neurological part within me held onto my early trauma. It was finally released when I allowed myself to talk about what happened.

Until my friend unwittingly created a safe space for me to share, I was afraid to talk about being smuggled out of the country. It made no logical sense. I had lived in the country for over two decades before sharing my birth story. I'd even become a US citizen. Yet the fear was real, and it was deeply embedded in my neurology. I did not feel it as fear. I just avoided it as my form of escapism. That past event perpetuated a strong sense of not feeling safe, one of many reasons why I stayed in perpetual action mode, whether that meant going out with friends, joining clubs, taking on projects, or learning something new—always driven to succeed. Part of the excess windy and fiery energy I carried stemmed from this early life trauma. I am grateful for its release, another step toward a more balanced state of mind, body, and spirit.

EARLY DEVELOPMENT AND STATE

Humans are born into an energetic state based on their elemental nature at birth, a state known in Ayurveda as prakruti, their birth nature.

The goal in life is to align with that birth state as much as possible, even if trauma is experienced, whether in utero, at the time of delivery, from a past life, or intergenerationally.

It is believed that the first sense of self comes from the viscera (the body). The connection to the stream of life is believed to be mainly through the gut. Your first sense of self comes from being able to register bodily sensations reflecting your experience.

In utero, nervous system development is fascinating. As the neuroectoderm (primitive) embryonic cells migrate upward to form the central nervous system (CNS), they also migrate downward to form the ENS, the nervous system in the gut.

There is no question that the gut and the brain are linked. The CNS and ENS come from the same embryonic tissue. It is no surprise that you feel emotions in your gut or that a communication link exists from the gut to the brain and vice versa. As the brain in your head begins to process sensory stimuli, the brain in the gut does the same. The gut feels things in a way similar to the brain.

As life progresses, adversity may draw you further away from your balanced state or prakruti to the imbalanced vikruti state defined by Ayurveda. This imbalance causes stress, which can lead to feelings of anxiety, sadness, irritability, or disconnect from self, among others. The gut senses these conditions. In response, it may become inflamed, leading to a sensation of queasiness or nausea; or it may spasm, leading to constipation.

When I struggled with insomnia during medical school, I was told I had major depression. I knew that wasn't my truth. My intuition told me there was something deeper the Western diagnosis didn't capture. The Ayurvedic diagnosis I discovered later embodied the mind, body, spirit, and social well-being aspects of my health, which conventional medicine completely overlooked. Ayurveda showed me I was energetically out of alignment. I now see it began with my early life experience in Uganda, and it compounded through the years.

Ayurveda identifies energy imbalance as excess in three states: windy, fiery, and earthy. These are related to the three mind-body (dosha) types discussed in chapter 1.

Windy/Vata Imbalance

A windy or vata excess triggers reactions similar to the freeze state.

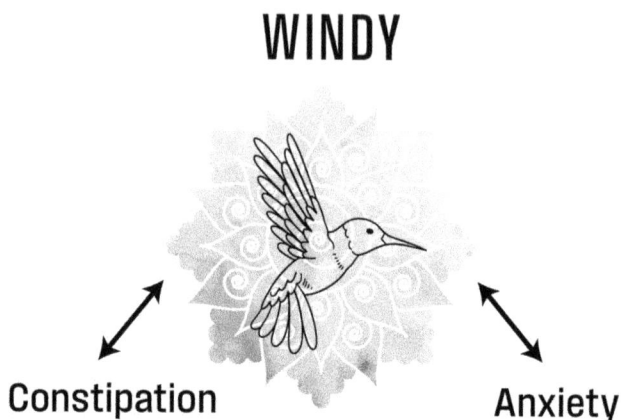

WINDY

Constipation   Anxiety

Fiery/Pitta Imbalance

A fiery or pitta excess triggers reactions similar to the fight state.

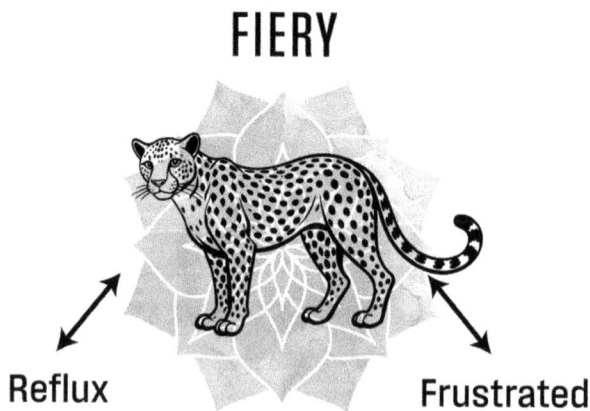

FIERY

Reflux   Frustrated

My struggle with sleep issues began with difficulty falling asleep, a vata or windy imbalance. This, along with skipping lunches, kickboxing, and drinking coffee, led to an additional pitta or fiery excess leading to challenges staying asleep. Heat started to emerge in my physiology, and I would become angry with life, my family, and even my bed!

Earthy/Kapha Imbalance

A kapha excess triggers reactions similar to the flight state.

EARTHY

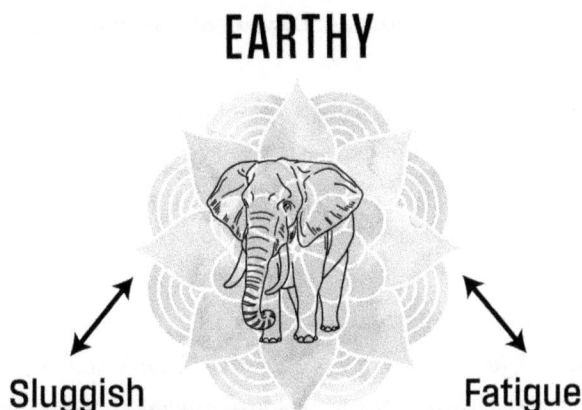

Sluggish   Fatigue

Eventually, my adrenals started to reduce their ability to keep up with this high-stress state. I started to drop out in cortisol production during the day and felt low energy, low moods, and low concentration. Thus, the diagnosis of major depression was given to me. This was my kapha, or earthy-appearing state, starting to show itself. I was depleted.

ADRENAL IMPACT

As you learned in the previous chapters, holding trauma for long periods of time overtaxes the adrenal glands. You may recall I found the majority of my patients suffered from adrenal fatigue, or as it's now known, hypothalamic-pituitary-adrenal maladaptation syndrome.

After testing numerous patients by having them perform four-point saliva cortisol tests throughout the day, I found that the majority had this condition. So instead of spending time, money, and energy testing, I began to confirm the diagnosis through the history provided by my patient or client and began treatments immediately.

These days, I believe many people struggle with an imbalanced hypothalamic-pituitary-adrenal circuit. Even more challenging, an imbalanced thyroid and hormone profile may be clouding the picture. The entire endocrine system is generally affected under stress or when trauma is held onto for too long. Low adrenal symptoms and low thyroid symptoms overlap.

Because this area is often challenging to address in the physician's office, I created a quiz, the endocrine assessment with focus on adrenal-thyroid axis, located at the end of this chapter. Although the quiz is by no means comprehensive, it lists the most common features apparent when an imbalance occurs. After you complete this basic self-assessment, please seek medical advice.

The quiz is for educational purposes only. Only start or stop treatment with the supervision of your medical provider.

Share your results and your thoughts with your provider and educate yourself further on these topics. Create a team that can support you as you clear the trauma from your mind and body and journey toward feeling optimal. You deserve to reduce the charge, clear that baggage, and live in your most authentically aligned state.

TAKE-HOME POINTS

1. Trauma is pervasive and has affected a far greater number of individuals than once realized.

2. Stress is common and involves the activation of the hypothalamic-pituitary-adrenal axis. With stress, your body can move out of

homeostasis.

3. Trauma leads to a change in your state, which can exhibit as a persistent windy (vata), fiery (pitta), or earthy (kapha) state, or some combination of the three.

4. When trauma is experienced, you develop a neurological part that retains a memory of the trauma. This part is in your subconscious and thus often not apparent to you.

5. Having a charge when discussing a story implies there is likely a part in your neurology that is holding onto a memory.

6. Clearing this baggage, or part, is helpful. It allows you to move back into harmony energetically.

7. Both stress and trauma can lead to an imbalance of your adrenal, thyroid, and hormone systems. Clearing the trauma improves the state of your endocrine system.

SELF-CARE TIME

After reading this chapter, evaluate whether trauma or stress has affected your endocrine system, precisely your adrenal-thyroid axis.
The endocrine assessment quiz that follows highlights the key features of adrenal or thyroid imbalance. It is by no means a comprehensive list of all the symptoms associated with dysfunction in these areas.

If you answer yes to one or more of these questions, consider following up with your provider to evaluate your adrenal and thyroid system fully.

1. Do you wake up with brain fog, feeling tired, unclear, or depressed? Or do you not feel awake until after 10 a.m.? _____

2. Do you have persistent fatigue, which isn't relieved by rest or sleep? _____

3. Do you find it difficult to handle stress, noise, or stimulation? _____

4. Have you felt overwhelmed and feel less productive? _____

5. Does your energy drop in the afternoon between 2:00 and 4:00 p.m.? _____

6. Do you have sweet/sugar cravings in excess? _____

7. Are you lightheaded or dizzy when you stand up? _____

8. Do you get a second wind after dinner? _____

9. Do you have pain? _____

10. Do you have cold hands and feet, constipation, dry hair/skin, or hoarseness? _____

Questions 1 through 9 apply to adrenal imbalances.

* If you answered yes to question 10, consider a thyroid evaluation with your provider.

This quiz is intended to empower you, to help you understand how stress and trauma may have affected you from an adrenal-thyroid perspective. Clearing the trauma and supporting these organs can balance these areas and have a powerful effect on your well-being.

7

Master Yourself

When Julie walked into our center, she was angry. Really angry. Rage flushed her cheeks and gave her a piercing glare. When she addressed my front desk staff, her tone threw them into a freeze state.

My office manager knocked on my door. "Julie won't be easy to talk to," she said. "She refused to get her vitals taken and said she wanted to talk to you right away about a medication issue."

I took a deep breath. "Please bring Julie to my office."

This was just one of many times I have worked with a patient who has gone into a state. As physicians, we need to understand that something triggered the patient. We shouldn't allow ourselves to take it personally, yet resisting that inclination is easier said than done. It is something I have seen and worked on for decades.

Going into a state is a natural stress response. I have experienced it myself. We all have. It's important to recognize what triggers you into a state and learn whether your state manifests as windy, fiery, or earthy. Once you can do that, learn to come out of that state as quickly as possible to avoid impacting your physiology. That is the trick.

Understanding this, I helped Julie come out of her state. By the end of her visit, she was calm and pleasant. This is an example of co-regulation.

CO-REGULATION

We learn how to manage state through co-regulation, meaning we rely on others to help us learn. As a young child, natural stressors would cause your system to shift into imbalance. If you were unable to move back into homeostasis on your own, you would look to your primary caregivers for help. If they had the tools and understanding, they would use tone of voice, soothing words, a gentle touch, eye contact, and body language to help you feel safe and draw you into their state, thus co-regulating you.

But for co-regulation to work, caregivers need the tools to soothe and nurture their charges. Whether they do depends on how well they were soothed and nurtured when they were younger. Eventually, through co-regulation, children learn to regulate themselves. But if your parents did not have these tools, you would have to learn to regulate yourself before your nervous system was fully formed. That's hard to do. If you were left on your own to regulate, as a teenager or young adult, you may have found yourself still turning to your parents, your significant other, your friends, or even your health care provider to regulate you.

There is a fine line between parental, friend, or spousal *support* and parental, friend, or spousal *co-regulation*.

One of the key aspects to healthy parenting (and healthy doctoring!) is giving someone the agency to regulate themselves. That's my goal with patients and coaching clients. I want them to create their own inner strength. When they do, they'll be their own best resources for health. When challenging situations occur, I allow them to experience the challenge, sometimes even fail in their response, and then grow from the experience. This is far more effective than pushing them to do things my way. In the aftermath of any failure, I do my best to counsel them about different paths available. Yet, in the end, they need to choose that path and experience it for themselves.

It is difficult to watch someone choosing the wrong path, yet creating room for them to find agency is important. When my patients and clients (and kids) stopped needing to consult with me because their symptoms resolved and they learned how to manage their system, I knew I had succeeded as a provider (and parent).

When patients continued to come in for treatment, I felt that I still had not done enough to give them tools to help them conquer their challenges. From a provider or parental standpoint, feeling as though we haven't done enough often causes a shift at the subconscious level, and we move from empathy and compassion into enabling.

Enabling

Enabling is doing something for another that they can do for themselves.

In the space of enablement, we may feel as though we're helping, but we are actually oppressing others and removing their agency. Enabling others tells them to ignore their inner wisdom and knowledge, thus preventing the development of intellect. Enhancing the intellect is similar to fine-tuning your inner GPS, your guide to navigating the adversities of life. If it isn't finely tuned, life will constantly present challenges, leading to pragyaparadh. A misaligned intellect is the number one reason we become sick, emotionally and physically.

Rather than enable others, we want them to build resilience and acquire agency.

Nonattachment

Nonattachment means staying neutral despite the outcome another person experiences, be it good or bad. The concept is challenging for many. When you attach yourself to another person—a child, parent, or spouse, for example—you lose your agency to act independently. Their happiness or sadness influences yours. If my daughter receives a poor grade, for example, she may feel angry and upset. As a non-attached parent, I would feel neutral toward her grade. That doesn't mean I wouldn't console her through a difficult time, it simply means her feelings do not become mine.

Ancient texts like the Vedas and the Bhagavad Gita show us that the concept of nonattachment has been a challenge throughout the ages. It's an ongoing one. I continuously work on nonattachment myself. From time to time, most of us will find ourselves attached physically, emotionally, and/or mentally, and we must embrace the process of independence—of nonattachment—as something to accept, not fear or push away.

Attachments

Attachments can be physical, mental, or emotional. Physical attachment may require being in proximity to a certain individual or even an object. These days, many people struggle with nomophobia—the fear of being without your phone. I have experienced firsthand the panic that arises when a phone goes missing, even for a few minutes! Emotional attachment may come from feeling happiness only when around another or doing a certain activity—like watching sports or eating chocolate, for example. Mental attachment aligns with your beliefs and views. You may be attached to a certain way of thinking, such as believing only medications can improve a health condition.

When you enter a group or family dynamic, are you still *you*, or do you blend into the group energy? Do you shift your personality to blend in? Do you have the ability to operate as yourself, where you can choose the best next step or pull yourself up after a challenge?

Or are you attached and codependent on one another to find guidance and balance? Parents need to co-regulate their children. Yet, at some point, they must allow their little chicks to fly from the nest and learn to regulate themselves.

You may even find yourself attached to certain koshas. You may attach to your physical body (annamaya kosha) and obsess about your workout or waistline. You may attach to your thoughts (manomaya kosha) and try to convince others of your viewpoints. These attachments are usually formed during your younger years when your brain is similar to a sponge, ready to absorb the thoughts, beliefs, and attitudes of your primary caregivers.

Damaging Belief Systems

My mother would often say, "Work hard. Otherwise, you won't succeed."

She said those words out of love and protection for me. They were based on her experience of being kicked out of Uganda and her desire for me to succeed, to find my place in the world. In response to that statement, I became obsessed with working hard from a young age. I even won an award as the hardest worker in my grade six class. While this work ethic helped me make my way into a top business school and eventually medical school, it was not without sacrifice. Like many others operating with this belief, I paid a price. I became very critical of myself and others. To prove that I could succeed, I pushed and studied intently so I could not perceive of failure—until I hit medical school, and insomnia stopped me in my tracks.

Any uneasy symptoms we experience are indicators of some form of stress. They force us to pause and evaluate our lives.

In the book *Stress and the Manager*, Karl Albrecht defines stress as:

A coordinated mobilization of the entire human body to meet the requirements of life and death struggle or rapid escape from the situation. The intensity of the stress reaction depends on the brain's perception of the severity of the situation.[1]

The key to this description of stress is the perception of situational severity.

What if you could shift your perception so that your system would not interpret challenging events as stressful?

As we have already discussed, early experiences have quite a profound effect on neurological programs and parts. These programs become hardwired into your neurology before you have a conscious awareness of them. My mother admitted she had a hard time saying, "I love you." She was unable to hug us or even accept physical touch herself. When she traveled with her friends to India, she did not want the daily massages her friends received. The truth is my mother was unable to be affectionate with us because she had a hard time loving herself.

Without self-love or the ability to accept it from others, what fills the reservoir? How could my mother express love to all of us when she had no love to give?

Even though you may not directly experience a traumatic event, you may be raised by generationally traumatized adults. My mother not only had the direct trauma of the Ugandan exodus but also inherited trauma from her mother and other women in her lineage. That is why the conversation about trauma is so complex and challenging. It isn't just what happens to us in this life, but also what happened to our parents in their lives and how our parents processed their experiences—or didn't.

Unfortunately, as I write this chapter, I am still processing the loss of my dear mother. I only wish I had understood how trauma affects all of us years ago. This understanding could have dramatically changed the course of her life and the diseases she developed due to the unresolved trauma.

Thus, it is my goal to share these teachings with as many people as possible.

The trauma of smuggling me out of Africa, losing her mother shortly after in a sudden car accident, along with any other trauma experienced earlier in life, most definitely affected my mother's egoic sense of self.

EGO, SENSE OF SELF, AND TRAUMA

Around age three, you begin to form your ego, or sense of self, and gain autonomy. This is based on Erik Erikson's stages of psychosocial development.[2] Without a strong sense of self, you seek approval from others. A lack of love, touch, and eye contact right after birth can have a lasting impact on your nervous system health.

During early infancy, the social engagement network forms. We learn to trust our environment and regulate ourselves based on social interactions. Calming voices and soft caresses from caregivers play an important role in neurological development. For more on this, read the work by Dr. Stephen W. Porges, *The Pocket Guide to the Polyvagal Theory*.[3] Without this sensory contact and left to their own devices, newborns can't regulate their nervous system when it gets triggered. Without intervention, this tendency can carry on into adulthood.

The concept here, again, is co-regulation. Your caregiver uses their tools to regulate and train your nervous system to find that calm, parasympathetic state. If this was missing when you grew up, you may find it difficult to soothe yourself and turn to external agents for support. This could be in the form of attachments to others, to food, to TV— you name it.

Many of my clients spend their lives seeking approval, love, and acceptance from sources outside of themselves, such as work, friends, colleagues, pets, kids, and, yes, even their medical providers. In my clinical practice, patients would often come in to receive love from me and my team, as they had an empty love bucket. This can be taxing for others. What you desire may be hard to fulfill. Love must start from within, so you are less in need to receive it from others.

When an acute traumatic event is happening and you are unable to run from it, you may find yourself going into one of three protective states: freeze, fight, or flight (dissociation). If the traumatic event continues to repeat itself or you hold on to the event emotionally or you hold on to the event emotionally, you continue going into state and quickly become stuck there. This explains how some people stay in a mode of windy (restless mind and contracted body), fiery (irritable mind and a heated, inflamed body), or earthy (depressed or heavy mind and a withdrawn, sluggish body) for most of the day.* This can lead to adrenal burnout and exhaustion.

Our adrenal system was meant to turn on for short periods of imbalance and then return to homeostasis, allowing us to feel connected to our baseline, authentic state. The adrenals are overtaxed when the system stays in a protective state for far too long. This is what some refer to as hypothalamic-pituitary-adrenal maladaptation syndrome and dysregulated adrenals and hormones. The internal rhythm of hormone production is lost, and it becomes challenging to maintain balance and healthy moods, sleep, and digestion.

---

*   See the Dosha Types on page 19 and 20 in chapter 2 of this book for more symptoms.

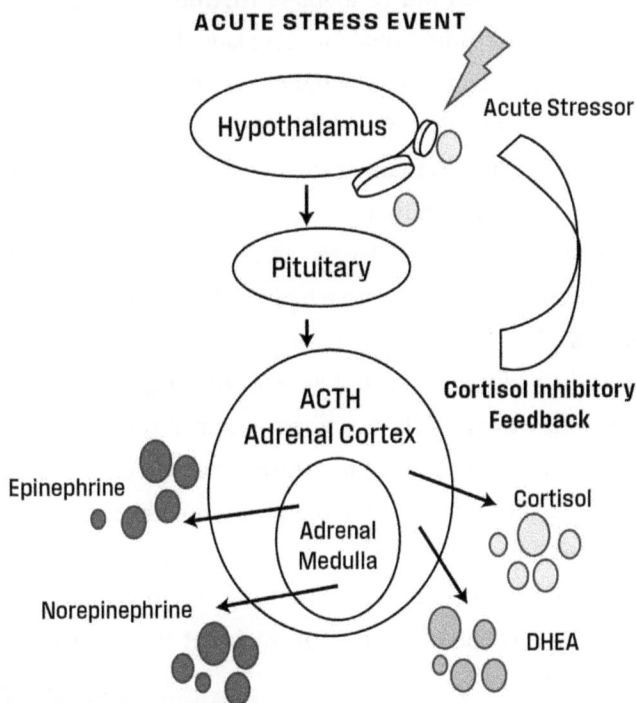

ADRENAL STRESS

ACUTE STRESS EVENT

- Acute Stressor
- Hypothalamus
- Pituitary
- ACTH / Adrenal Cortex
- Cortisol Inhibitory Feedback
- Epinephrine
- Adrenal Medulla
- Cortisol
- Norepinephrine
- DHEA

If you feel unable to speak about a particular situation, express your thoughts, or speak freely around certain individuals, you may be experiencing a prolonged stress response. When stressed, the blood flow shifts away from Broca's speech area of the brain and toward your muscles to help you escape from danger. Digestion slows down, and libido vanishes. Hormones shift into fight or flight instead of rest and repair. How could anyone be interested in sitting down to eat a turkey sandwich or having sex when a bear is chasing them? No wonder there are so many fertility issues in the United States these days!

Stress causes another key shift: avoiding eye contact with others. Looking away allows one to stay inside themselves and avoid interaction with a world perceived as untrustworthy or unkind. Voice and tone of speech may change when feeling unsafe. Facial expressions such as anger, disappointment, sadness, or fear are often readily visible.

Trauma pushes us out of a stable rhythm to enter a triggerable state. It perpetuates more imbalance and launches a vicious cycle leading to a state of disconnect. It happens so subconsciously that we are not even aware of the disconnect. Friends and family notice we are not as responsive by phone, email, or even text. We go into state. The egoic self blends into a personality that is not really us. This protective state tries to move us away from danger. Eventually, we visit the doctor to find out why we are having stomach pains, headaches, or not sleeping, for example.

This is the body telling us that we need to realign with self.

Think of the triggers we described earlier. Trauma and triggers are directly related. When something upsets you, especially when it upsets you more than others around you, there is likely trauma—a.k.a. baggage—lurking underneath it. Baggage consists of the unprocessed feelings and thoughts about an unsettling situation that occurred in the past with another individual or an event that overwhelmed the nervous system.

Imagine you were driving on the highway and enjoying some of your favorite music. Out of nowhere, a car side-swiped you. You lost control of the vehicle and spun off the road. After that event, you may have believed you were fine, as you sustained no physical injury. You shook off the event, believing you got over it.

Yet later, when cars drive close to you on the highway, your heart races or your palms grow sweaty. There may be a subtle entry into a windy state as cars pass. Your neck tightens, your hands grip the steering wheel, and your stomach churns. Even talking about driving on the highway or listening to the song that played while you were driving could bring you into state.

It's incredible what the subconscious mind holds onto from previous traumatic events. The goal isn't to ignore the traumatic memory and pretend it doesn't exist; this could worsen it. Instead, it's better to accept how you go into state and learn how to clear that program from your system.

Post-traumatic stress disorder evolves from traumatic events that are not cleared. Unfortunately, reminders of the trauma lead to a state of hypervigilance. Such a traumatic memory often does not naturally clear on its own and tends to worsen over time unless addressed with coaching or other tools.

TRAUMA AND YOUR BRAIN

Remember the amygdalae, the two almond-shaped structures in the deep, limbic brain that store memories of trauma? The amygdala is very perceptive to the environment, always scanning for danger. It may, at times, detect danger when danger is not present.

I believe the amygdala is in direct communication with the sub-conscious mind and subtle body, areas that hold onto the emotions and thoughts of an earlier dangerous situation. The amygdala may overreact to a situation simply because its memory of a similar situation overrides the current danger. In this way, it picks up on nuances of another person's eye contact, body language, and even their style of dress, to create an internal representation before the person has even spoken. This internal representation may be in alignment or imbalanced based on the baggage carried in the amygdala (and the subtle body). A disproportionate, trauma-heightened response may result, simply because these clues serve as a reminder of someone who acted or appeared the same way and caused harm.

It is hard to be in the present moment when you are always living in the baggage of the past, isn't it?

The medial prefrontal cortex (mPFC) controls the activity of the amygdala. That's the part of the brain that lets you know if previously threatening individuals or situations are safe. For those with a history of trauma, the connection between the mPFC and the amygdala is not strong. Under trauma situations, the mPFC dampens down, and the limbic and reptilian brains take full control of you.

Holding onto trauma or baggage is unhealthy for several reasons. First, it keeps you in a reactive mode. You go into state far more easily than you should. Second, simply having a history of trauma affects the hippocampus, which is involved in learning and memory. For example, if I walk down an alley as a young child, I may not have any negative impression of it. Yet if I had walked down the alley with my mom, and she warned me to stay near or someone could attack me, I would probably be nervous the next time I walked down the alley. Traumatic events, or even words, can create a memory we may hold onto for years.

The beauty of the nervous system is something called neuroplasticity. This means that your brain can remodel itself. With various exercises and techniques, you can strengthen your brain, similar to working out a muscle in the gym.

Many smaller triggering events—from a problematic interaction with a friend to a challenge at work or eating poorly—can add up. These microaggressions inflict small yet mighty insults to our system. Eventually, those microaggressions overflow, causing a reaction to something minor, such as your child not doing his or her chores. With no visible reason, you explode with anger.

Bingo. You have baggage.

People commonly believe that a problem from the past has been resolved, even when it affects them in the present. Reactions triggered by past trauma are normalized and accepted as part of who they are. This normalization allows further suppression of trauma. Often, there is stigma around trauma, so many choose not to accept it or do not want to discuss it. That, too, only makes the trauma worse.

It is fascinating how thoughts and physiology that protect us early in life become the thoughts and physiology that imprison us in the present.

Many people undergo therapy or other self-help work such as journaling. While these tools can be helpful, keep in mind this idea: the more you talk about the negative experiences you have had or currently have, the more you anchor them as your truth. It becomes tough to move out of trauma when you focus on what went wrong versus understanding the message behind the challenge and growing from it positively.

So, look for the message.

I often tell those amid a difficult situation to remember things always seem hardest right before major shifts happen. Once you realize that challenge allows the greatest growth, magic can happen for you.

CAUSES OF TRAUMA

Clearly defined traumatic experience examples:

- Divorce
- Car accident
- Sexual abuse
- Emotional abuse
- Bullying
- Being mugged
- Pandemic
- Being abandoned
- Not being loved
- Death of a loved one

Collective traumas—those that affect all of us as a collective:

- Pandemic (Spanish flu, polio, COVID-19)

- Climate change
- War
- Natural disasters
- National news (murder of JFK, 9/11)

THREE MAIN TYPES OF TRAUMA

Trauma can be classified as acute, chronic, or complex.

1. Acute trauma results from a single incident.

2. Chronic trauma is repeated and prolonged yet may not be interpersonal (such as living in a violent neighborhood or experiencing ongoing harassment).

3. Complex trauma is repeated or a series of negative event that takes place over months or years. This usually begins in childhood and is often interpersonal in nature (childhood abuse, neglect, or bullying).

SYMPTOMS OF TRAUMA

Here is a list of common symptoms that may be experienced with trauma:

- Hypervigilance or being excessively "on" or triggerable
- Shock, denial, or disbelief
- Confusion, difficulty concentrating
- Anger, irritability, mood swings
- Anxiety and fear

- Guilt, shame, self-blame

- Withdrawing from others

- Feeling sad or hopeless

- Feeling disconnected or numb

- Intrusive thoughts of the event that may occur out of the blue

- Nightmares

- Visual images of the event

- Loss of memory and concentration abilities

- Disorientation

- Confusion

Just like Arjuna in the Bhagavad Gita, a great warrior in the moment of conflict chooses to fight instead of surrendering and laying down arms. The key to mastering yourself is to avoid surrender. Get to understand your nature, who you are in balance, and who you become when you go into state. Then, dig into what triggers you. Look for the trauma underneath it. Release the grip this past event has on your current well-being. When trauma is cleared and the neurological part that holds the memory softens, you will become less triggerable over time. Connect to your physical body and begin to move into the subtle body. The easiest way to do this is with the breath, as discussed in earlier chapters.

Once you release past trauma, you will see how much healthier, happier, and connected to yourself you become. Familiar but hurtful stories disappear, and you learn to see things as they are. The false lens of the personality that has been protecting you will fall away.

You may even find yourself stopping to smell the roses.

The goal of this chapter is to help you understand that you can, indeed, master your state by learning about the trauma that shapes it. For the best results, consider working with a trauma-informed coach or therapist.

We all carry trauma, whether large or small. No one is immune to it. Experiencing the COVID-19 pandemic was traumatic for most people. Clear the baggage from your trauma and strengthen your nervous system so that you can regulate yourself in a balanced fashion. Your ultimate goal is to respond to threats appropriately and turn off the stress response easily when the stressor has ended.

In this way, you can return to homeostasis, moving out of state and into bliss.

TAKE-HOME POINTS

1. Co-regulation occurs when you utilize other individuals to bring you back into homeostasis.

2. Enabling occurs when you repeatedly do something for another that they can do for themselves.

3. When someone enables you to continually co-regulate through them, they prevent you from fine-tuning your own inner GPS or intellect. This leads to pragyaparadh.

4. Physical, mental, and emotional attachments prevent you from developing resilience.

5. Stress is linked to the *perception* of situational severity. If you can shift your perception, you can shift your stress reaction.

6. Trauma can be passed down from one generation to another. This is referred to as generational trauma. Pairing that with a lack of sensory connection to a parent or primary caregiver when you were a child can worsen your trauma profile or baggage.

7. The biggest challenge with trauma is that the situation occurred in the past, yet it affects your present. This likely moves you into one of the three states: windy, fiery, or earthy.

8. Acknowledging that trauma exists and working with a health

care or wellness provider to clear it can have a profound impact on your well-being.

ACTION STEPS

This self-care journaling exercise can help to identify what triggers you.

Start by practicing the reverse nostril breathing exercise described in chapter 3. Consider using a calming essential oil to turn off your reptilian brain and quiet the amygdala. Scents are very individualized. Try out a few and find your favorite. I love vetiver, eucalyptus, and camphor for grounding and opening my nasal passages. You can place a few drops on your wrists and third eye to help deepen your practice.

Caution: Always test a small area of skin with one drop of oil to be sure you can tolerate it. Also avoid putting the oils in your eyes, mouth, or any open cavity.

Then, grab a journal, examine the trauma list provided in this chapter, and answer the following questions:

- Is there anything on that list you have experienced that may have led to trauma for you?

- When you shift into state, are there any links to early trauma?

- Have you discussed your trauma with anyone else—friends, therapist, coach, or doctor?

If this exercise provokes strong feelings, thoughts, or emotions, please consider reaching out to your provider for support in this area.

8

Taking Ownership

"It is just not fair," Molly said as she sulked in her chair.

"What is not fair?" I asked.

"Why am I the only one who can never find the right guy?"

As often happened during my clinical visits, the conversation quickly shifted from the medical complaint that brought Molly in to see me to a session focused on life's challenges.

When I start probing into why the patient or client struggles with sleep issues, anxiety, pain, or a whole host of other symptoms, I often find myself moving into a conversation about career challenges, dissatisfaction with relationships, and the challenges of being a spouse, parent, or child. My medical assistants are instructed to knock on my door if I run past thirty minutes for a routine follow-up visit. How do you finish a conversation about job dissatisfaction or relationship troubles when you realize that you've discovered the root of someone's ailment?

Needless to say, they would knock at my door quite often.

I love having these conversations. They allow me to evaluate a patient from a unique perspective versus solely seeing them as someone with just medical symptoms. I embrace delving into the nuances of how my patients and clients live.

Why do they feel stressed? Why are they unsatisfied and unhappy with life? Whom do they blame? Themselves or others?

The answers always lie far beyond the symptoms and the original diagnosis. I often tell them a lack of connection and happiness within the self led to the disease, not vice versa. If we work together to find the cause of internal imbalance, we can make a stronger and more positive impact on disease.

As I explored the topic of having a life "that was fair" with Molly, I thought about a brilliant speaker I heard on YouTube: Michael Beckwith of the Agape International Spiritual Center.[1] I found his words beyond powerful. He discussed four stages of spiritual evolution:

1 **To Me** → 2 **By Me** → 3 **Through Me** → 4 **As Me**

Stage One: **To Me**	*Stage Two*: **By Me**
I believe something outside of me determines my fate. I am a victim.	I can use my mind to create my life and take responsibility for it. I am a manifester.
Stage Three: **Through Me**	*Stage Four*: **As Me**
I have done enough inner work to recognize life happens through me if I allow it to. I am a channel.	The line of separation between me and all life has dissolved and I feel at one with all. I am it.

Your mind gradually reaches a better place as you move through the stages. If you get stuck in victim stage, life remains challenging. When responsibility is extended to external sources, power is also given to those sources.

A similar idea is expressed through the Japanese concepts of *kensho* and *satori*. Both explore the nature of growth. The former symbolizes growth through challenge and pain, while the latter symbolizes a sudden and profound experience of enlightenment or awakening that provokes growth without pain.

Kensho is the Japanese word for "seeing one's true nature." In other words, seeing things as they are. We all have kensho moments in life. Sometimes these moments begin as challenges, something difficult to face or accept. If we view their occurrence as an encouragement to pause and shift trajectory, we can begin to see the truth.

Pain + Personal Growth = Kensho

Insomnia inspired my kensho moment. My life was completely off-balance, and insomnia allowed me to wake up to my truth. If I were in spiritual stage one, as Dr. Beckwith described, I would be asking, "Why did this insomnia happen *to me*?" This aligns with the "life isn't fair" conversation and the victim mindset.

As I read some deep and compelling books during pivotal times in my life, I began to move into the second spiritual stage of satori, asking, "Why is this happening *by me*?" stage or "How am I manifesting this?" I began to understand the meaning behind my symptoms and ask what I needed to change or shift in *me*. By doing so, I accepted responsibility for my situation—and reclaimed my power. Once I shifted in this direction, everything in my life shifted.

I have witnessed the same shift in countless others. Once it begins, fewer kensho moments occur, and if they do, they are less challenging to manage.

Ideally, we move from kensho into satori. Satori moments allow enlightenment, growth, and evolution without pain or struggle. Satori moments are the goal.

One of my favorite quotes frequently attributed to Viktor Frankl, the author of *Man's Search for Meaning*, is: "When meaning is given to suffering, it ceases to become suffering."[2]

Your symptoms are not the problem. Your symptoms are likened to the smoke of a fire. The fire is the problem, not the smoke. The goal is to discover the root cause or core issue (the fire) beneath the symptoms (the smoke). Put out the fire, and the smoke disappears. Find and conquer the core issue and watch symptoms resolve.

Whether they understand the full impact of stress on their lives or not, most people refer to stress routinely. In my early days, I did not feel stressed because I had become accustomed to being "on" all the time. That was the only state I knew.

One of my Ayurvedic trainers checked my Ayurvedic pulse, similar to Chinese medicine practitioners, to evaluate my well-being. He asked me what I did in my *off* time. I realized, at that moment, that my *off* time was just as hectic as my *on* time. How would it be possible for my adrenals to reset and recover?

You may be in the same state that I was in. Maybe you never really turn off or recharge. In this scenario, if you have symptoms yet do not feel stressed, it may be best to consult another who knows you well. They can help you understand how your stress reveals itself through your language, actions, and behaviors. They can even take the stress personality quiz with you. Often, others can see you better than you can see yourself.

You may be able to distinguish your stress state from a non-stress state. You may say certain scenarios or situations allow you to feel stressed, your boss or mother-in-law stresses you, or you notice stress more when you have not slept well.

It is interesting to evaluate how stress became part of your vernacular.

FOCUSING ON THE WHOLE SELF

The ancients believed people were spiritual beings having a human experience. Mind, body, and spirit were not separate entities. They were all part of what made us human. As a result, approaches to health involved balancing our mental-spiritual side. The approach was holistic and systems-based, with the mind and body working as one entity.

Spirituality was linked to physical health until philosophers like René Descartes tried to separate the mind and body. Gradually, the public began to question if the mind and body operated independently or in unison.

Does the mind control the body?

Does the body affect the mind?

Should religion or spirituality be part of a health care discussion?

In 1802, at the end of the French Revolution, medicine and religion were officially separated.[3] When, some 130 years later, the discovery of penicillin eradicated the bad bugs causing disease, the mind and spirit were left completely behind. The wellness focus shifted toward the physical aspects of symptoms and disease. This reductionistic and fragmented approach assumed that organs and systems operated independently, without any connection to each other. Instead of harmonizing the human system to create balance and coherence, health care concentrated on fighting off pathogens and eradicating the symptoms of distress.

When I suffered from insomnia, the purely medical model rooted in these shifts gave me a diagnosis and a prescription that left me feeling unheard and misunderstood. As I tried to explain the sleep challenges and my curiosity regarding the onset, the physician tried to align me with a "checklist" of symptoms, to fit me into a specific diagnosis, and thus, a precise remedy.

I only wish it were that simple.

One drug working on one neurotransmitter or peptide hoping to fix the complex problem at hand is quite a task to achieve. There is no question medication can improve symptoms. That is what is to be expected. It is simply not possible to have long-lasting, complete eradication of symptoms by using only this approach. Humans are intricate beings who rarely present with a simple condition. At the time of my diagnosis, I was seeking a deeper answer that reflected on the health of my mind, senses, and spiritual self, not simply reducing my symptoms.

I wanted to get to know myself.

*"It is far more important to know what person the disease has
than what disease the person has."*
—Hippocrates

As we discussed before, ancient Ayurvedic wisdom offers a more holistic view of health. So, health is a state where the tridosha (constitutional nature), digestive fire, all the body tissues and components, and all the physiological processes are in perfect unison and the soul, sense organs, and mind are in a state of total satisfaction and content.

Taking the time to honor symptoms when they arise and address them early truly reduces the burden of disease and the cost of health care. Spirituality in medicine is now showing promise as more evidence is suggesting how adding a spiritual component may lead to improved longevity[4] and even a reduction in inflammatory cytokines along with depression.[5]

Unfortunately, despite growing evidence of the impact of spirituality in health care, it is still often forgotten in the doctor's office. Too much focus is placed on making a diagnosis and reducing the symptoms. It doesn't help that visits are time-limited and the patient expects immediate alleviation of discomfort. The entire model must shift from the doctor to the patient to honor this way of approaching health. Understanding the person (or environment) is fundamental to improving any condition. While I am grateful for the new medicines available for acute conditions such as infections, along with managing chronic diseases such as cancer, disabling migraines, and autoimmune disorders, our society must not forget the importance of utilizing these medications in an environment that is receptive to them.

If I try to grow a plant in poor soil, the plant will likely not grow well. If instead I choose soil enriched in nutrients and keep the soil moist, the plant will grow nicely. The human body is similar. Taking a cholesterol medication while continuing to consume an unhealthy diet will reduce the medication's effectiveness. The same happens with the mind. Constant stress and worry that a medication or treatment will not work creates an unhealthy environment, and it likely won't work. This is called the nocebo response—a self-fulfilling prophecy. We can negate the benefits of the medication if we have lost hope that we will get better or believe the medication is not powerful enough. This has been proven time and time again.

Why not shift your program so you can believe not only that medications will work for you but also your life wishes will be fulfilled along the way?

Your mind is so influential toward health that it even plays a role in how you process food. In the "Mind over Milkshakes" study, researchers measured the ghrelin response of participants who were given a milkshake and told it was either "indulgent" or "sensible." Ghrelin stimulates the appetite. Those who drank the "indulgent" milkshake were found to have a reduced ghrelin response—meaning they felt fuller—than those who drank the "sensible" milkshake. Think about that. It was the same milkshake, yet the body had a different response based on the perception of the mind.[6]

FOOD AS MEDICINE

Many believe that Hippocrates was the father of medicine. He aligned with the belief "let food be thy medicine and medicine be thy food."

According to Ayurveda, the physical and emotional bodies are tied together. There is very little separation, as they influence each other. Food carries a life force known as prana. Not only does your mind interpret the food, as the milkshake study indicates, but the food also affects your mind.

One of the most powerful proverbs in Ayurveda is:

Without proper diet, medicine is of no use.
With a proper diet, medicine is of no need.

Food is powerful in Ayurveda. Based on your nature, foods may balance or disturb your energy state. Similar to humans, foods carry the five elements in different proportions. Foods are categorized as vata-, pitta-, and kapha-balancing or vitiating (unbalancing) based on their composition of elements. Leafy greens, when eaten cold, for example, vitiate (unbalance) the vata dosha due to the high proportion of air elements in their nature.

The elemental nature of food is key when using diet to balance out your stressed personality.

Meal Timing

In addition, the time of day you eat plays a role in your health. Aligning your meals with your circadian rhythm truly has an impact on your mind, along with your microbiome—the 100 trillion microbial species in your gut and all over your body.

The concept of timing is based on the patterns of the sun and moon. It is believed that your biggest meal of the day should be eaten when the sun is at its peak, at noon. At this time, you generate the highest amount of digestive enzymes and hydrochloric acid. Dinner should be no later than 7:00 p.m. As the sun sets, enzyme and acid production fall. Thus, having a large meal at 8:00 p.m. may not be digested well.

Lunch used to be the biggest meal of the day. In the United States, this shifted, according to Sarah Lohman, a culinary historian who wrote the book *Eight Flavors: The Untold Story of American Cuisine.*[7] For more information on that topic, I would highly recommend her book.

The importance of eating and living in alignment with the circadian rhythm has been recommended for thousands of years. This alignment with the daylight cycle is known as *dinacharya* in Ayurveda. Dinacharya rituals include getting up at the same time each day, having lunch as your biggest meal, eating dinner by 7:00 p.m., and going to sleep around 10:00 p.m. nightly. Following these principles help us feel connected to the cycles of the sun and balance the HPA axis.

We tend to be more insulin-sensitive early in the day. That means muscles are better able to absorb and utilize glucose from the bloodstream. Thus, eating lunch as the biggest meal has been clinically proven to be helpful for weight control. Studies now confirm that eating dinner later in the evening leads to the inhibition of an enzyme known as hormone-sensitive lipase. This is an enzyme that helps release fat from your fat cells while you sleep. Eating a late dinner may inhibit this hormone, thus making it more challenging to burn fat and regulate blood sugars. In addition, late dinners are linked to an increase in cortisol (stress hormone) production.[8]

This novel area of research, known as chrono-nutrition, is not truly that novel, as eating in alignment with the circadian clock has been taught in Ayurvedic literature for thousands of years. I am grateful many are realizing the importance of timing meals versus simply focusing on what is on the plate to create improved body composition, regulate blood sugars and cortisol, balance hormones, and even shift mental and neurological health.

The importance of aligning with the circadian rhythm and maintaining optimal health was studied by researchers who won a Nobel Prize in 2017 for their work on this topic. The prize was awarded to Jeffrey C. Hall, Michael Rosbash, and Michael W. Young for their study of the molecular mechanisms controlling the circadian rhythm. They studied fruit flies and found they contain a gene that controls the normal daily biological rhythm. The gene was shown to encode a protein that accumulates in the cell during the night and is degraded during the day.

This discovery gave evidence of a biological clock inside the cell. The clock regulates hormones, sleep, body temperature, and metabolism. What they found was fascinating. If there was a mismatch between the external environment and their internal biological clock, this led to an increased risk of various diseases.[9] This work, proving that *not* following the circadian pattern increased disease, won them a Nobel Prize.

Ancient wisdom is truly being proven by modern science.

Seasonal Impacts

Another food factor that affects your health is seasonal changes. Foods shift in abundance during different times of the year, as should the foods you consume. This is challenging when a wide variety of foods are available in the local grocery store, even when they're not in season. Mangoes, a tropical fruit, should not be abundant in Chicago in January.

Ideally, eat what is in season and rotate your diet as the season changes. Eating foods in alignment with the season supports microbiome health. Microbes on foods change from season to season, as does your microbiome.[10]

Modern science is proving what ancient medicine like Ayurveda said five thousand years ago. This wisdom is not only part of the Ayurvedic system, as many great thinkers and other systems of healing had similar revelations. It is simply packaged differently.

START WITHIN

Many ask me for the secret Ayurvedic tricks to weight loss and longevity. I do have a few tricks up my sleeve, yet the truth is it starts with working with your mind and then honoring your diet. Start by reducing the battle within and figure out what is at the root of your conflicted mind.

Some people look at food as their enemy. I used to look at my bed as my enemy. I would feel angry at myself when I could not sleep. The moment I started to view insomnia as the tough-love messenger letting me know I was disconnected from myself and my truth, things shifted. I practiced acceptance and allowed myself to be uncomfortable with discomfort. I allowed myself to believe that there was a reason for my challenge.

It is said that there are moments in your life that will define you. Moments that, at the time, seem inconsequential. My struggle with insomnia was one of those moments. It would take me years to understand this idea of a transformational moment and the concept of kensho. I have now come to realize that when these kensho moments happen, they stop you. You have no choice but to pause and reflect.

I had lived a good life, yet one with such drive and intensity I had never taken the time to pause and reflect on my *why*. I never even gave myself a chance to get to know myself. I was too busy moving to think. I spent time outward and rarely went within. I had no idea who I was or where I was going. I simply knew that I felt uncomfortable if I wasn't doing something every moment. Staying on and active allowed me to feel productive. Yet, in the end, I realized that rushing ahead without insight into who and where you are headed only leads you to feel stuck, unhappy, and unsatisfied.

Are you feeling disconnected? How do you get unstuck and out of disconnection?

It starts with creating inner harmony. Once you create inner harmony and take ownership of your thoughts, words, and actions, serious shifts happen on the outside too—and they can happen quickly. I am beyond grateful that I never took the Prozac and instead chose to explore the kensho experience, to look for why my experiences were happening *for* me, not *to* me.

The main focus should be on understanding *why* the kensho happened and what the message is behind it. If you can start to embrace the *why* behind discomfort, you can begin the journey to resolve it. Even though you may believe that you do not have choices in life, you do. Every moment of every day offers you opportunities for choice. Yes, your initial choice of thought or action may be generated at the subconscious level. I get that. Your system—based on the sensitivity of your amygdala and the baggage it and the subtle body carry—may habitually move you into a freeze state when someone speaks to you in a certain way. The voice or tone of an individual may remind you of that disrespectful partner you dated in your teens. In this state, your neck may spasm, your colon may constrict, and your mind may feel anxious. The initial entry into state may be at the subconscious level, yet at some point, you will become aware that you not only entered but are staying in state. At that point, you must find tools to exit that state as fast as possible.

Why, you ask?

The reason is simple. If you stay in state for too long, you overtax your adrenals. That is the setup for symptoms, disconnection from self, and, eventually, disease sets in.*

For example, staying in a windy state leads to excess vata, which can create a freeze state of mind-body-spirit. The goal is to move back into a homeostatic state after the stressor is over rather than staying in the state for hours or days after the event.

WINDY

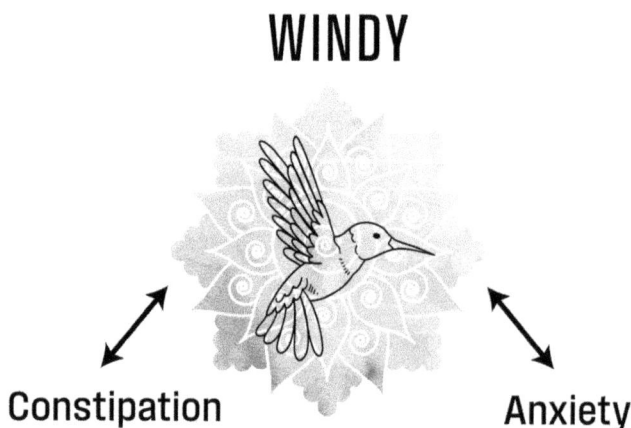

Constipation   Anxiety

You must first recognize that you moved out of your baseline connected state in the first place. This is the challenge. It takes time, as most people live in a disconnected state unless they worked on connecting with the subtle body.

---

* For more information about how disease states occur, see *The Mysterious Mind*, chapter 8, "Vata Dosha: Move Like the Wind," chapter 9, "Pitta Dosha: Rage Like Fire," and chapter 10, "Kapha Dosha: The Dosha of Groundedness."

I say this with all my heart, as I was that person years ago. Only after forcing myself to pause and reflect on my life as challenges occurred—a.k.a. kenshos—could I become more able to recognize when I shift out of alignment. I now know myself well enough to know when that happens, and I can catch myself earlier and move back into balance with the tools I have acquired over the last two decades. When I get triggered into a state, I evaluate what part of me got triggered and work to clear that charge. I still have a way to go, yet the process becomes easier the more I practice it.

> *"It is not up to you what you learn. It is merely up to you whether you learn through joy or through pain."*
> —Marianne Williamson

MOVING BACK INTO HOMEOSTASIS: THE CONNECTED STATE

When it comes to taking ownership, this, to me, is the most important part: taking ownership of yourself.

Owning your thoughts, your beliefs, your attitudes, your words, and your actions are key. We live in a time with access to tools to help us investigate why we think, act, and behave in a certain way.

Statements such as "my mother was like this" or "I have this condition because it is genetic" no longer garner sympathy. Using excuses is not taking ownership. That is laying blame on your parents or your genetics. You now have enough data to support the impact of mindset, diet, and lifestyle on disease manifestation. True, if you had a parent with healthy genes and fantastic athletic skills, you are more likely to be capable of playing sports and avoiding the doctor. Yet, the reverse is not true. My mother had migraines, and I do not. My father had high cholesterol, yet my cholesterol is normal.

Spend some time reflecting on your struggles and remember to embrace the imperfect life. Ask yourself, *what gift does this bring to me?*

In a time of struggle, ask, *why this is happening for me?* instead of *to me?*

A challenge often reflects the universe's invitation to evolve into a higher level or version of yourself. It is time to grow and learn versus becoming the victim of your story.

9

How Resistant Are You?

Resistance is natural. It is not unusual for people to rebel when they realize their early childhood programming—the hypnotic theta brainwave pattern that governs behavior—does not align with their truest self. Eventually, if they rebel and have the tools, they move into a more authentic version of themselves, which brings a greater state of bliss. However, that shift can often be difficult to make in the face of external world pressures and expectations.

Back in the day, no matter how much yoga I did, or how many supplements I consumed, or how many lifestyle changes I had made, I often felt challenged to find my own bliss. I checked my labs and found that my thyroid peroxidase (TPO) antibodies were through the roof despite optimal results for other labs. These antibodies indicated my body was creating an immune defense system by attacking my thyroid gland. Yet, other than an elusive grasp on bliss, I felt perfectly fine.

It was 2007, and I was embarking upon an incredible journey of opening a wellness center with a partner. The center was divine. After pouring energy, time, and money into the space, we transformed it into the gorgeous center we had visualized, complete with a yoga studio, ample massage rooms, a lovely apothecary, and an inviting team of practitioners.

At that time, I operated the North Shore Headache Clinic within the wellness center. It was a bit challenging to run the clinic, mainly focused on migraines, while codirecting the center. It made sense to do so, however; all the wellness center offerings would benefit the patients I was serving. The center gave me plenty of tools to help bring my own antibodies down.

Yet something was missing.

When I referred my clients to other practitioners or modalities, a curious thing happened. Some of them started coming in more frequently to see the other practitioners while continuing their visits with me. A few patients improved. They reduced their visits and treatments. However, the majority found little change to their underlying condition and still requested their monthly Botulinum toxin type A injections and an array of supplements to keep their system in balance.

The same puzzling condition held true for my antibodies. Even after taking many supplements, having weekly massages, practicing yoga, going gluten-free, and removing my mercury fillings (the latter both recommended by my integrative circles for TPO antibody reduction), my antibody levels stayed high. This is not to say the other modalities were not helpful. They certainly were. I just felt something was missing in my health care toolbox.

I now realize that the missing tool—for my patients and for me—was a focus on the subtle body. We received beautiful and helpful treatments from the most talented practitioners without fully healing the imbalanced subconscious program. This program, lodged in the subconscious mind (SCM) and hidden in the subtle body, maintained a state of imbalance. Often, even with some improvements, disrupting life events would completely derail progress.

Soon after this realization, I slowly began incorporating meditation into my personal daily practice. I studied mantra meditation, a practice that allowed me to focus on a specific sound or phrase to quiet my mind. After a few months of diligent practice, I felt more present and reflective. I began to honestly examine myself, asking who I was and what I wanted in life. I focused on my dharma, my life purpose. During this time, I cleared more of the baggage stuck in my SCM by learning NLP and practicing hatha yoga, which involved deeper breath work.

After this focused effort, *everything* began to shift. My practice grew tremendously, I was asked to appear on national TV multiple times, my speaking engagements flourished, and I was thriving in my personal life. Eventually, my TPO antibodies came down too.

I had finally found that missing piece, and I shared it with my patients.

Why did daily meditation have such an effect on me? And can it have an effect on you?

Meditation soothes the default mode network (DMN) and internal ama, or toxicity. To fully understand how this works, let's take a closer look at the DMN.

THE DMN

The DMN is a complex network of brain structures that includes the posterior cingulate cortex (PCC) and the anterior medial prefrontal cortex (aMPFC). The DMN consolidates your memories and experiences to form associations between them that help life make sense. In fact, it is linked to your inner dialogue, or what you say to yourself, which is based upon the MOW behind your perspective.

The DMN is the brain's default mode. It's where thoughts go during periods of wakeful rest, when your mind wanders, or when you engage in mindful activities such as meditation. The DMN automatically takes over when the brain is not involved in externally oriented, cognitively demanding mental tasks such as accounting or figuring out a problem at work or even concentrating on cooking a meal. It's also where you go when you take a quiet walk along the lake or meditate.

A healthy, balanced DMN gives the brain time to rest while

promoting beneficial memory integration, mind-wandering, planning, self-reflection, and emotional regulation. It will also switch on and off easily between wakeful rest and cognitive tasks. When the DMN is working properly, it lowers the risk for mental health issues. In many ways, the operations of a healthy DMN are like healthy sleep, when a series of chemical processes cleanse the body and mind and consolidate information. Dreaming, specifically reaching REM sleep, is believed to be essential to emotional processing and emotional memory consolidation.

On the other hand, an unbalanced DMN can wreak havoc. Instead of letting the brain rest, the DMN becomes overactive. It prevents being fully present and on task for life's demands and from appreciating the simple joys of life. And to create further imbalance, if the DMN is overactive, it can lead to an overactive mind at night, thus impacting sleep. This can create a vicious cycle.

An unbalanced DMN perpetuates a negative inner dialogue that can sabotage efforts to live a fully engaged life. An impaired DMN consumes attention and energy, imposing a greater risk for physical or psychological disorders. Studies by Marcus Raichle and Abraham Snyder in 2007 show that upward of 90 percent of the energy consumed by the brain supports the DMN.[1]

Three Directions of an Unbalanced DMN

Based on some impressive research, the brain tends to operate in one of three directions while the DMN is turned on.[2]

1. Others: You may start focusing on the beliefs, intentions, desires, and perspectives of people other than yourself.

2. The past: You may begin to dwell on previous events—situations and circumstances you cannot change.

3. The future: Alternatively, you may worry about events or encounters that haven't yet occurred.

These three directions are aspects of excessive self-referential thinking. In other words, thinking about yourself in excess. When your mind wanders and you start to daydream, instead of being in a quiet, receptive, and creative state, you go into past events and plans for the future or think about what another person has said or done to you. Rumination points back to the concept of ama, the internal baggage lurking in your subconscious mind that needs to be cleared.

Reducing the activity of the DMN is now being linked to a reduction of disease. There is clear evidence proving that patients with depression have a more engaged DMN.[3] The brain focuses on negative perceptions of themselves and the world. Often, during times of engagement, the individuals with depression can only focus on themselves instead of paying attention to the desires and needs of others. This is not to lay blame; it is not the fault of someone struggling with this disease. It is more to understand the power of the DMN and how it can hijack the brain from a state of calm and rest. In addition, research has shown that an overactive DMN is linked to diseases such as dementia, Alzheimer's disease, and schizophrenia.[4]

Theoretically, when the DMN is in the rest state, your brain should utilize fewer resources than when you are engaged in an active task. The fascinating new research on this area reveals that most people shift to overly engaging the DMN at a higher level. Thus, the brain truly never turns off to consolidate and reset. When the DMN is engaged in excessive self-referential thinking—in other words, out of balance—it is impossible for it to enter the imaginary, creative, and intuitive mode it was designed for.

Imagine what that does to the HPA axis and your cortisol levels! When one stops moving and performing tasks and the brain enters into DMN activity, the nervous system remains tremendously active, maybe even more active than when performing tasks. This may further activate the adrenals versus allowing them to rest.

Role of the aMPFC and PCC

Within the DMN network, the aMPFC and the PCC brain structures communicate with the temporal lobe, specifically the hippocampus.

Why is this important?

If you remember from earlier chapters, the hippocampus is the home of memory. Memories are key to life experiences. Pleasant memories often take us back to times of happiness and peace. Unpleasant memories may give us feelings of sadness or anger. Unfortunately, these negative memories often resurface during periods of stress. Recently, when I encountered a few nights of poor sleep, my brain reminded me of that time of insomnia, and that memory brought the programming from those days back to my conscious awareness. I hadn't thought about sleepless nights in years, yet there I was, lying in bed, recollecting every emotion and thought I had experienced during those troubling times. Thankfully, this time I had the tools to shift my brain program and move back into a solid sleep pattern.

As you can see, the DMN can take us to places we do not wish to go, back to traumatic events. It can even create a story about our lives that may not be true. This story appears for many of those I work with who state they are lonely. Loneliness is a subjective perception of social isolation, which means there is a discrepancy between what is actually happening and what individuals perceive.[5] Loneliness, one of the biggest challenges many individuals face, may cause them to say yes to too many social engagements, spend too much time on social media, or even work excessively for fear of going home and being alone.

Loneliness is linked to a 29 percent increased risk of heart disease, a 50 percent increased risk of dementia, and a 32 percent increased risk of stroke.[6] Add to that, loneliness is now linked to excessive DMN activation. Individuals may believe that they are alone in their challenges, not supported, or simply not included. Yet, research shows the DMN creates this story when it may not reflect reality. For further understanding of the DMN, feel free to read the review by Daniel S.

Barron, PhD, and Stephanie Yarnell, MD.[7]

MEDITATION CALMS THE DMN

To overcome my TPO antibody challenge back in 2007, I slowly began incorporating meditation into my daily practice. I started to get introspective and ask myself who I was and seek my dharma, my life purpose.

When I have spoken about the power of meditation, the typical reaction is the belief that meditation seems very difficult to do. When I ask why sitting quietly for two to three minutes daily is difficult, the response is that it's too hard to turn off the brain, as once the brain is quiet, a multitude of thoughts enter.

When you have trouble reaching a calm, peaceful state of meditation, ama has accumulated in your mind. For many of you, meditation seems like a daunting task, as you are unable to quiet your mind even for short periods. I cannot even begin to explain the multitude of beneficial effects quieting (and clearing) the mind has on your physiology.

Accessing the DMN in this way allows you to connect with a side of you that is blissful.

You begin to make sense of your life, your path, and your reason for being here.

The DMN, when in harmony, may be likened to the anandamaya kosha, or bliss layer of your subtle body. Your true self.

Unfortunately, when the mano- (mind) and vijnana- (intellect) maya koshas ruminate over thoughts and beliefs that may not serve you, you may not be able to reach anandamaya kosha. Your true, ideal self is free of the programs of the past, future, and who you are *supposed* to be. It is who you are at the core.

Do you see why it is good to connect with it once in a while?

Recognizing an overly activated DMN is imperative to move into harmony. Unfortunately, many do not. They may even enable this center, thus hardwiring the pattern.

BUILDING RESILIENCE AND CONQUERING RESISTANCE

As I noticed my resilience growing, I realized those who were able to conquer their pain shared a key element to success. They were building resilience by developing tools to improve themselves. Similar to a parent who longs to help their child, we were unintentionally enabling our patients at the integrative center through their reliance upon injections, medications, acupuncture, massage—you name it. In a way, I was enabling myself too, by expecting external support such as massage, supplements, and a strict diet, on their own, would shift me (and my antibodies). Yet the tests showed that approach alone was not working.

Why was that happening?

It would take me stepping away from that practice and starting Zira Mind and Body Center to realize the truth of what I was missing. Only when my patients and I did not have as many external tools did our deeper journey of self-discovery through mind and spiritual work begin. I am grateful for this discovery!

If your thought program keeps you with a MOW that says life is stressful, and you are alone and lonely, for example, no matter how many supplements, yoga classes, or massage sessions you utilize, you will still rely upon external regulators of your nervous system to feel safe and secure. Depending on the specific supplements, type of yoga, and massage you incorporate, you may nudge the subtle body gently. Yet, the truth is it takes a concerted team effort to truly improve the subtle body and reprogram the SCM, along with balancing the activity of the DMN.

At that time, which was around 2007, my MOW still had me convinced that I needed to be busy to be successful. I kept introducing new tools, new supplements, new integrative testing options, and new lectures—all of which kept me in a state of continual wind and fire excess. My MOW stood in the way of system self-regulation and harmony.

In a way, this is similar to the co-regulation associated with parenting. A healthy parenting model co-regulates with children so that when they reach a certain age, they can regulate themselves. For example, if your child falls off the swing, you do not ignore them and keep talking to your friends. Nor do you immediately panic and rush over in a reptilian mode, which would make them feel they are in danger. Instead, you acknowledge the fall, and as long as it was not a severe incident, you swiftly yet gently walk over to check in on them. You give the child a chance to process their state and create their own reaction to the situation. You do not create a reaction for them, which would imply you are regulating their emotions on their behalf. The goal is to co-regulate *with* them, not *for* them.

In a way, when symptoms occur, lab tests go awry, and we become fixated upon repairing the problem with supplements, lasers, acupuncture needles, and even yoga poses, we give the responsibility for healing to an external source. We allow the modalities to tell us what will be. I am a big fan of many of these modalities, yet herein lies the key point: these tools must be used alongside subtle-body work with clear goals in mind of what you and your provider want to achieve. The intention must be clear from the onset. You must evaluate your thinking and feeling patterns, reconnect with your breath body, and fine-tune your discriminating center—the vijnanamaya kosha—so you can choose the best things to support your deepest, most balanced self.

Do not forget about pragyaparadh, the mistake of the intellect, as the number one cause of disease. Instead of relying on external sources for guidance, we must trust our own innate wisdom.

Strengthen your intellect and succeed in all areas of your life. It should be easy, right?

Yet why is this SO HARD to do?!

What keeps you from taking ownership?

Resistance and Ego

Resistance is real. It's more common later in life after certain viewpoints and beliefs have become fixed, locking in a certain pattern of thought that even the intellect can't overcome. When the DMN is over-activated, those locked patterns of thought create emotional barriers to resilience, or egoic blocks.

The ego is formed in younger years to give you a sense of who you are and what you are meant to do in this world. Often, it doesn't have a chance to form fully as others—especially parents, friends, or religion—influence who you think you are. For example, I met a parent recently who told me her daughter loved basketball. When I spoke to the daughter at another time, she told me that her mother forced her to play because it was her mother's favorite sport in high school. The daughter didn't care much for the sport. Over time, if the daughter continues to succumb to her mother's view of who she really is, she will develop an egoic block. She won't be able to act upon her own desires for fear of disapproval from her mother.

In that scenario, you can see how the ego of the parent influences the ego of the child.

As parents, we must be careful not to project our desires, wishes, and unmanifested dreams onto our dear children. They are meant to live their own lives, not ours. I try to remind myself of this daily. It is not easy, yet this is the only way they can form a strong sense of self, leading to a strong sense of agency, which is an ability to advocate for themselves.

People naturally become more resilient when they know who they are and what they want out of themselves and their own lives. I meet many people who say, "I should have," or "I would have." Dreams or wishes are unmanifested as they choose a life that their parents or society deems is the right way to live versus the one meant for them. Instead of building resilience, they build resistance.

If you've ever felt uninspired or experienced a lack of drive, the reason is likely simple: you are tangled in resistance. You are resisting the life that someone else wants you to live and, at the same time, resisting the decision to live the life meant for you.

Resistance can occur in other ways too. When I meet someone who says, "I will never do yoga," I often inquire where that resistance comes from. At times, it comes from fear. Fear of the unknown or being uncertain may lead to resistance. I am amused by how many people say they "can't do" yoga. Yoga is more about balancing and connecting with the mind than it is about perfecting a downward dog posture. Yoga develops a connection with yourself through breath, gentle movement, and quieting the mind. It is meant for everyone to practice, not a select few.

It is natural to lean toward a feeling of security and safety. When you do not feel safe or comfortable in a situation, such as eating a new food—or something even more common, public speaking—you may resist. But resistance imbalances you further and keeps you stuck.

Think about what led you to choose staying in the safe zone.

Are you only doing things you are comfortable with? Or limiting yourself from living in any way?

Saying, "I can't," or "I will never," is a reflection of your ego's health, your sense of self. This may reflect your sense of self-worth.

Pain is another reflection of an attempt to escape the world you live in. No one chooses pain, yet pain comes to help you distance yourself from disharmony within. Instead of retreating to your room during a migraine, ask yourself what in your life is not aligning with your true self. Pain invites you to wake you up and stop hiding from your truth. Instead, move into it. Ask yourself what the meaning of the pain is and how you can evolve from it.

Think about what you do to avoid pain and why you choose to avoid it in that way.

What keeps you from taking ownership of the situation behind your pain?

TAKE-HOME POINTS

1. Resistance is natural. It results from a mismatch between your neurological program and the one that was passed down to you generationally or through your parents.

2. The DMN is considered a "default" network, as it is where your brain goes when it is not engaged in externally driven tasks. It is referred to as the "default" state because it is linked to the mind in a rested, consolidative state where we move into imagination, creativity, and intuition.

3. Two of the key brain structures comprising the DMN are the posterior cingulate cortex (PCC) and the anterior medial pre-frontal cortex (aMPFC). These two regions are connected to the hippocampus, your memory center. Memories of past events or situations may keep you engaged in a particular circuit of thinking.

4. Ama, or baggage, often leads to excessive DMN activity. Excessive DMN activity is linked to diseases such as Alzheimer's disease, depression, and schizophrenia.

5. Your ego is your sense of self. The ego can become attached and lead to excess in DMN activity. Resistance occurs when you are in this attached state.

6. Being attached to your thoughts, beliefs, and/or even your physical body can prevent you from being present for your external tasks and the needs of others.

7. A healthy ego represents a healthy sense of self. You are resilient and have agency to advocate for yourself and your desires.

SELF-CARE TIME

In yogic philosophy, various methods are utilized to subdue the mind. Asanas, or yoga poses, are only one method to relax a stressed mind. Another approach employs the idea of candle gazing, known as *trataka*. This practice moves you into an immersive experience that allows you to step away from your thinking mind and train your DMN to enter a more balanced physiology.

During this practice, your goal is to keep your eyes open and control involuntary actions such as blinking. Start with short intervals and stop if your eyes burn or tear up. This practice builds concentration, helps clear the mind of negative thoughts, and calms the mind.

Technique: Obtain a candle. You may even choose one with a calming scent to enhance the experience. Sit in a chair. Place the candle at eye level, about an arm's length away.

Close your eyes and focus on the spot between your eyebrows to settle your mind. Then, open your eyes. When your eyes are relaxed and focused on the candlelight, gaze without blinking.

If your eyes start burning or tearing, feel free to close your eyes and rest.

If able, try the technique again, repeating three times, one minute each if possible. Build up so you can gaze up to ten minutes without blinking.

A beautiful technique to refresh the eyes after practice is to rub your hands together, generating heat, then place them over your closed eyes. Rinsing eyes with cold water may be helpful if the eyes are burning.

Keep practicing and notice the effects on your mind.

10

Discovering the Self

"Work hard or you won't succeed."

My mom shared that mantra repeatedly during my younger years. As a child, with my sense of self not fully formed, those words sank into my brain circuitry. With no ability to resist, they programmed me to have a particular viewpoint and belief system, one shaped by hers. After we left Uganda to start a new life in Chicago, that work ethic and mantra helped my family survive. My mother loved me, and she shared those words to protect me according to her view of the world, which was shaped by tragedy.

That mantra had a powerful effect on my behavior. I focused every moment on the goal of achievement. Through the years, I watched my mom sacrifice her life to get ahead. I was not about to live my life in vain. I wanted her to be proud of me. I wanted my life to have a purpose. I wanted her to know that her sacrifice had meaning and would not be forgotten.

Academically, I excelled in all classes. Beyond the classroom, I picked up tennis in grade school and became a varsity tennis player in high school. I started babysitting when I was eleven years old. At the age of fifteen, I found my first employment at McDonald's, even though couldn't legally obtain a worker permit until I was sixteen. I dedicated myself to filling every break in my schedule with work, even though my family was financially stable. I even secured two jobs the summer before my first year in college. With every break in college, I worked, rarely taking a day off.

For me, working meant far more than earning money. I felt safe if I worked. It gave me an internal sense of value and worthiness. It also fueled the false belief that success only comes from hard work—working to the point of little time for anything else.

Hard Work = Success: True or Not?

A strong work ethic did earn me a spot in a top business school and medical school, yet those opportunities did not come without a price: the challenge of insomnia triggered by stress. *When the demands placed on the organism exceed the organism's ability to handle them, the organism begins malfunctioning.* While I was in medical school, stress led to adrenal dropout, a.k.a. hypothalamic-pituitary-adrenal maladaptation syndrome (say that quickly three times!). In today's terminology, this would be considered stage one of adrenal burnout. I had barely begun training, yet my mind pushed me to physical exhaustion.

At the time, I battled internally with the external choices I had made. Deep down, I believed the Western model of medicine didn't suit my perspectives. I only went to medical school to satisfy my egoic need for acceptance from the Indian community I grew up in. Even though my father was a physician, I barely understood what a physician did. I had never needed one growing up. My father took care of any medical exams and paperwork necessary for schools and sports, and I was blessed with good health.

As evidenced by my initial consultation with the psychiatrist, some misalignment during the early phase of medical school led to sleep issues. I didn't think I belonged there, yet I had been accepted to a school where so many of my peers wanted to be and had not been given the opportunity. *How could I leave? What would I do with my life? People would be so upset with me if I left,* I thought. *They might even mock me for not being able to handle the workload.*

I was occupying a spot in a coveted medical school program without appreciating my good fortune. Those who longed to be there in my place, along with other friends and family, would question my sudden desire to leave. Additionally, I was fortunate to have parents who paid for my education. Education was of prime importance to them; it would help me survive in this dog-eat-dog world. Education would help me make something of myself and succeed in life. It felt like a worthy investment.

With so much going in my favor, I often thought I should be grateful and get over my hesitation.

Confused and overwhelmed by my situation, I asked Mom if I should leave medical school. In a calm and rational voice, she told me if I wasn't happy, I should leave, but I suspected she was thinking, *I told you so!* You see, my mother had told me *not* to go to medical school. She based her rationale on the length of training, which would interfere with my ability to have a family.

I wasn't ready to sacrifice my career for a family. I witnessed first-hand how Mom suffered from giving up her love for teaching and students after we were forced to leave Africa. Instead of returning to the classroom as a home economics teacher, she focused her energy on her family, cooking incredible meals while raising three daughters and a cousin who lived with us. She had loved teaching, and she missed it. She encouraged me to work hard so that I would have the opportunity to get a good degree and a job that would satisfy me.

How sad that Mom's first job in Chicago was a midnight shift at Motorola. She put gold plates on beepers to make ends meet while my father repeated a residency program in internal medicine—this, after practicing medicine for years back in Africa. Humbling times, to say the least. She never gained the momentum to find employment again. She sacrificed her passion and her happiness to raise us and take care of my father.

Mom was beyond talented in the art of cooking, and her heart was filled with love and service. Cooking for others became her profession. She loved doing it, yet I believe she held herself back from serving at an even higher level. She dreamed of opening a catering business. It never happened.

Unwilling to let my desires go unmanifested as my mother had, I pursued medicine. During my episode with insomnia, I wasn't sure if I could continue. I told Mom that if I didn't pass my anatomy exam that week, not to pay the tuition bill. Despite my desire to succeed, to follow my dreams, I was exhausted and ready to leave. She told me there was no shame or guilt with that choice. It was vital for me to be happy. If I left, all would be fine.

As you might guess, I passed the anatomy exam.

This memory brings tears to my eyes, as I recently had the same conversation with my daughter. She chose to leave a coveted computer engineering program in her college to pursue industrial engineering. Industrial engineering, while a challenging program in itself, was not quite as difficult to get into as computer engineering. Although the switch might seem like an easy decision, it created tension for my daughter and my husband. He firmly believed that computer engineering was her golden ticket to a life of success, a common belief in our community. How could she leave such an opportunity after working so hard to get in?

The turmoil played havoc on her immune system. Just as I had trusted my instincts and decided against Prozac for insomnia all those years ago, Ariya trusted her intuitive voice. She shifted to a direction more in alignment with her soul's calling.

It wasn't easy to step away from computer engineering, yet she did, and she now thrives in industrial engineering. I am grateful we had the tools to guide her at that moment of conflict. If I hadn't experienced a similar conflict myself, I likely wouldn't have guided her this way. I am grateful she spoke her truth and followed her wisdom.

How do you live in alignment with your true self?

How do you follow your own truth versus the truth of others?

You must escape your illusions, or in Sanskrit, your *maya*.

ESCAPE YOUR MAYA

Many people live in a world of maya. It's like a mirage, something they believe to be there, yet isn't. This world of illusion arises from programmed patterns of belief and behaviors. Do you ever wonder why you are not healthy? In an unhappy marriage? Unsuccessful in your career? At a subtle level, subconscious programming leads to a life that is not harmonious with who you really are. The best way to wake up to reality is to liberate yourself from your egoic way of living and thinking.

Remember the movie *The Matrix* and the choice between the red or blue pill? Liberation comes down to choice. But it's challenging to make the best choice when your thinking is clouded and led by your imbalanced personality, your *false self*. The false self, the self that is not the real you, is often defined as the ego, yet it is more than an identity associated with self-importance or self-esteem. Rather, it is a constructed sense of personal identity associated with external factors. The false self emerges as the person we have been programmed to believe we are.

The mind is divided into four parts known in Sanskrit as *buddhi, manas, chitta,* and *ahamkara*. Buddhi is the intellect, which operates with the information or data you have collected over time—and only that information, creating limitations. Manas is the mind, as in the sheath known as the manomaya kosha, which we discussed previously. Chitta refers to the cosmic intelligence. This is the knowing derived without prior actions, knowledge, or memories. Ahamkara is the ego or sense of identity. Ahamkara is derived from the Sanskrit word *aham* meaning "I am," and *kara,* meaning "doing."

When you are aligned with your ego, your life aligns with your desires and how you want to show up in the world. An imbalance in your ego creates a false self, leading you into a predominance of one of the three stress personality types—vata, pitta, or kapha. This is where issues arise. This is when your choices do not align with your true self but instead, the desires of your personality. Life becomes a series of missteps leading you off course from the final destination to your soul's ultimate happiness.

How do you balance your ego?

What is getting in the way of your success in life and ultimate happiness?

It is a journey. For now, I ask that you reflect on your current state and learn which stress personality is giving you imbalance.

EGO AND ATTACHMENTS

Remember the importance of healthy ego development. Your ego must truly align with your deepest self, not one influenced by the goals and desires of those around you. Recognizing which part of your ego has been influenced by others is key. When the ego is imbalanced, it begins to form attachments with a wide array of external desires to substantiate its identity. These can range from material possessions, relationships, and social standing to physical appearance, power, pleasure addictions, and more.

The attachment of your ego to external desires is one of the biggest challenges you face. They pull you out of harmony. A stable egoic nature helps you understand who you are, why you get out of bed each morning, and how you show up in this world. Yet, unfortunately, the ego gets clouded by attachments. These attachments may be generated by programs you have inherited from others. They keep you stuck in the very behaviors that led you toward them!

Achieving a state of connection with your true self can only occur after you clear your fears and detach from as many desires or attachments as possible.

This is challenging to do in today's world. Imagine going a week or even a day without technology—no phone, computer, or TV—while trusting that your family and work are taken care of. How would you do? Could you let go? If you cannot imagine this scenario, your ego is attached. Your sense of self depends upon managing the conditions impacting family and work. However, to be healthy, you must form and maintain an ego that needs nothing outside of itself to feel whole.

When your five senses receive incoming signals, your brain decides which ones to cue into and which to delete because you cannot attend to the two million bits of information presented to your nervous system every second. You choose the 126 bits that are relevant to you and your needs at the time. Attachment occurs when you are drawn to certain sensory experiences and have a challenging time disengaging with them. You may be attached to certain foods or drinks. You may be attached to your spouse or child. Your sense of self and identity slowly become established around these attachments.

Attachment Examples

Years ago, I had a client who was attached to M&Ms—the candy-coated, button-shaped chocolates. Although she was serious about her health and took many steps to improve her well-being, she could not kick her attachment to her afternoon M&Ms. The M&Ms gave her a sense of happiness and joy in the middle of her workday and setting that aside was a severe struggle for her.

You could be attached to a visual input such as Netflix. It is easy to get attached as one episode ends and the next automatically begins without having to lift a finger. Maybe you love crime shows, and you can't stop watching them. You may be attached to certain kinds of music, such as intense rap or hip-hop. Remember the imprint of your sensory body on your subconscious program. If you habitually employ external mechanisms such as eating sweets, indulging in crime shows, and listening to intense rap music for some form of relief—practices that activate your reptilian brain—your system will move into a more reptilian, imbalanced state versus a relaxed prefrontal cortex brain program.

If you aren't sure if this is what you're doing, consider this question: *if you go a day without it, how do you feel?*

Your ego gets attached to senses or material things, such as your work or identity (I am a doctor, for example), and you lose the essence of who you are.

Some patients have a hard time calling me by my first name when they meet with me for the first time. I greet them by saying, "Hi, I am Trupti," instead of, "Hi, I am Dr. Gokani." That may be an unconventional greeting for someone visiting a board-certified neurologist, yet I want us to meet on an even playing field. I want to set the tone of collaboration, of working together. Too many patients want their doctor to fix them. I view my role as someone who will guide and educate yet never fix anyone. "Fixing" has to be something someone does for themself. I want my patients to become their own healers after working with me.

With this perspective, being a doctor did not become part of my identity. I am secure enough in myself and my skills that adding "Dr." to my title adds no value to me, it does not make me feel more worthy or intelligent. This also allows my patients to feel more vulnerable and connected with me as a person who also struggles with life, not as their doctor who seems to have it all figured out.

There are many ways to assess whether the ego has attachments. In my practice and now coaching, I often recommend doing a seasonal cleanse. This is one of the longevity-promoting practices in Ayurveda and many other systems of healing. Fasting and cleansing are wonderful times to test your attachments and reset your mind and body. Over the years, I have been surprised by the number of attachments I've discovered. Staying away from the item of attachment for five to ten days has an incredible effect on the mind and body. For example, it is liberating to not *need* a cup of coffee or even a workout each morning yet consume or engage with it simply because you enjoy it.

Forgive me for being blunt, but many of you have a sense of self that is attached to your family, your work, your car—you name it. When another individual or item has become part of your identity, the resulting attachment creates problems for achieving harmony in your soul. When I closed Zira Mind and Body Center, that integrative neurology center I had spent fifteen years building, I felt a profound, indescribable loss.

I was surprised by how much closing the clinic affected me. I had sent kids off to college, moved away from my parents, shifted career paths, and lived in different cities, yet closing the clinic was particularly traumatic. You see, the center had become a part of *me*, part of my identity—even though being called "Dr." had not. When friends and family asked me what I was doing after the clinic closed, I was at a loss for words to explain my path. I had developed a wonderful coaching program in place of the clinic and recruited many beautiful clients. I knew the program allowed me to work at a much higher level than possible in the clinic, thus it had the potential to be more fulfilling, yet part of me identified with being an owner of an integrative center. Suddenly, with that center gone, I felt as though a part of me was missing.

The clinic was an attachment.

Thankfully, I allowed myself to be uncomfortable with the uncertainty of where life would take me. I delved into my new coaching program while reconnecting with myself, my husband, family, and friends. I pursued writing this book, read the Gita with a study group I formed, and started a yoga certification course.

Releasing Attachments

When it comes to attachments, we all have choices to make. Even though they may be partially subconscious, if we pay attention, we have a conscious recognition that we choose these things repetitively to give us a sense of happiness, however fleeting. Notice the word *choice*. We have a choice. We can choose to not become dependent on external items to fulfill or complete us. The goal is to feel content and peaceful at all times, whether these external items are present or not.

Of course, many of us love going to concerts or movies, eating delicious food, or receiving a loving call from someone we care about. The problem occurs when we *depend* on these things to keep us happy. If we derive happiness from externalities, it may become difficult to achieve a stable sense of contentment and happiness internally without them.

One of the most effective ways to clear attachments is to surround yourself with the ideal support network as you shift toward strengthening your ego. Who do you choose to expose yourself to?

I chose to surround myself with people I loved who supported me on my journey. Then I took specific actions to enhance my growth. Eventually, I was able to disconnect from my attachments and rise above them. When I no longer felt the need to define myself with the integrative center, I began feeling a sense of completeness within.

Unfortunately, if you are attached to a sensory experience—or an item that leads to a sensory experience—it takes awareness that you have an attachment along with a gentle reduction of exposure to that item to balance your egoic needs and stabilize your personality.

To balance your ego, refer to the ego quiz at the end of this chapter. Explore the health of your ego, determine what attachments you carry that aren't serving you, and release them. Think of it like organizing and cleansing your home to make it feel welcoming and balanced. Doing a little housekeeping around your attachments will ultimately create balance in your DMN.

Attachment Centers

After looking at your sensory attachments, you can then move into evaluating the three areas where your attachments lie: your body, mind, and intellect.

1. Body: An attachment to your body, the annamaya kosha, occurs when you are overly focused on your appearance or physique. Do you spend most of your time thinking about how you look or how your body performs? If so, you may be attached to your body in an unhealthy way. There is a fine line between caring for your physical body and obsessing over it. Spending hours at the gym to have the perfect arms at the expense of quieting your mind and understanding why you are feeling unhappy is not an ideal investment of your time.

   While it is important to eat healthy foods and perform occasional cleanses, relationships with either can lean toward the extreme. I have had clients who went into a full-on panic if they ran out of supplements or forgot to take them for a few days. In the majority of cases, this will not make a difference. Obsession with appearance, exercise, and nutrition are all manifestations of attachment to the physical sheath.

2. Mind: Your thoughts, the manomaya kosha sheath, can also become attachments. Maybe instead of spending time on your physical body, you focus on the internal chatter of a voice that constantly worries, criticizes, judges, or simply comments on every aspect of your life. Some refer to this as the inner monologue, as we discussed previously. This is part of the DMN. It is quite common to have an inner monologue, yet getting attached to it is a different story. One of the biggest challenges with my patients and clients involves disconnecting from their inner voice. Most of the time, this voice is negative (often parental!), thus the attachment to this chatter perpetuates further imbalance in the self.

3. Intellect: The last attachment area concerns the intellect or inner knowing, the vijnanamaya kosha. Attachment here is associated with an ideology or more universal beliefs. For example, if you have an attachment to a religious group or political belief that

is excessive, this can lead to an imbalance in the system. It is fine to have an interest or preference for a belief or viewpoint, yet having a dogmatic attachment and inability to see another perspective is where trouble occurs at this level.

The Inward Nature of Attachments

Attachments may influence you to turn inward, which can become problematic. Some of you may be so inwardly attached that you have become selfish. You do not choose selfishness; it simply happens as the false ego grows stronger. If this is you, you tend to be self-indulgent and self-important or the opposite—self-loathing and self-pitying. The conversation is always about you and your own good or bad situations in life. When others talk to you, the discussion centers around you.

Does this sound like you?

Take a hard look at yourself. We all have the capacity for this state, especially with life's inevitable challenges around parents, kids, work, friends, and so on. It is important to have supportive friends with whom you can share grievances to simply get them off your chest. Yet if the majority of your conversations revolve around you and your life situations, your ego may be out of balance. The DMN becomes overly engaged in the mental processing of your self-referential thoughts. It is difficult, in this state, to even think about other individuals or obligations at work or home.

If you cannot enter a group and quietly listen to others, this may be an area you need to work on. Begin by taking a deep breath and acknowledge that this imbalanced ego is only formed to protect you. Your system believed you were in danger and thus began pulling away from the danger, moving inward. With such inner absorption, there is no space or time for anyone or anything else.

Therein lies the problem. With an egoic imbalance, you may tend to delete others from your life. They may choose to delete you too.

RELEASE YOUR ATTACHMENTS

You can only release your attachments if you recognize them. One way to do that is by consciously connecting with your nervous system. Neuroception helps you do that. My goal, after training in neurology, is to help you develop a keen sense of the way your nervous system coordinates your bodily functions, responses, and sensory experiences. You want to become so perceptive of your nervous system that if its activities start moving out of alignment, you quickly become aware and shift yourself back to baseline. In this way, you are constantly fine-tuning your nervous system to work harmoniously for you.

Clearing your attachments and balancing your ego allows your nervous system to become resilient. It's similar to calming a newborn. After exiting the cozy womb, the newborn may initially require swaddling with a blanket, a pacifier, and gentle rocking motions to fall asleep. Eventually, the swaddle may go, yet a pacifier or rocking may still be required for the infant to drift off. The goal is to eventually remove these external supports and allow the newborn to reach a deep slumber on its own. By doing so, the newborn learns to trust their internal signals and release appropriate sleep hormones, thus leading to a restful night of sleep. Eventually, newborns feel capable of soothing themselves and know sleep will happen naturally.

If dependency upon the pacifier—or the parent—persists, this attachment can prevent the nervous system from fully developing. The newborn becomes insecure about being able to do this process alone. The ego and sense of self start to form during this time. Self-reliance at this early age determines the ability for resilience in the years ahead.

The ego represents confidence that you can navigate life and determine your path on your own and guide your system to live life in alignment with your true self, aligning with the cycles of nature. This is the premise of ancient wisdom. In this state, you can live in the most harmonious, happiest way in mind, body, and spirit.

Balancing your ego is a journey. For now, I ask that you reflect on your current state. Determine which personality or Vedic type—vata, pitta, or kapha—is creating imbalance. What is getting in the way of your success and happiness? Achieving a state of connection with your true self occurs after you clear your fears and detach from any desires and attachments.

ANALYZE YOUR SOUL: ATMA VICHARA

Atma vichara is one of my favorite concepts. *Atma* refers to the soul, and *vichara* means deliberation or analysis. It is the idea of analyzing your soul. It means going beyond the thinking mind of who you are and allowing an inner knowing to give you a sense of who you are. The challenge here is that you cannot use your mind to figure it out. We must pause to hear that inner knowing speak. We simply cannot hear it unless we are still. To get silent and observe, your DMN must be in balance.

See how this all comes together?

As Ayurveda revealed how disconnected I was and how to achieve the connection I needed, I felt compelled to share it with my patients, my family, my friends—with the world—so others could learn about it too. Without hiring a publicist or doing any marketing, I was humbled and grateful to be invited as a guest on Dr. Oz's show in 2014. This was quite an honor, considering I had zero media training and had never appeared on national television. At the time, this show had about ten million viewers. Colleagues of mine had been waiting for years to get on the show. I suddenly felt as though the universe was telling me it was time to share my message with the world.

I presented insights about dosha typing, and it was a success! I am amused that my mother-in-law thought I would be making *dosas* (Indian crepes) with Dr. Oz versus talking about doshas. We had a nice laugh and then I launched into the meaning of doshas.

Even though my mother-in-law was raised in India, she was not versed in Ayurveda. Ayurveda was not accepted in India until 1970 under the Indian Medicine Central Council Act.[1] Now, the WHO and other organizations are making efforts to globalize and standardize the practice of Ayurveda. With thousands of years of practice behind it, Ayurveda is finally being accepted into the mainstream.

As I helped others discover their truths, I began to feel that most Ayurvedic dosha quizzes were not helpful. Most people do not recognize where they are imbalanced. It's difficult to see yourself clearly when your body is operating at a subconscious, somewhat hypnotic level. As they say, it's hard to see the forest for the trees. If the patterns were conscious and obvious, you would change the program and course correct.

If it were only that easy.

Imagine wearing the same pair of glasses year after year, even as your vision weakens. Things grow blurry through those glasses; you may even feel off and get headaches from them, yet you are used to seeing and feeling that way. When you visit the ophthalmologist and don the newly prescribed lenses, suddenly things become clear. Though it may take a brief period of adjustment, your mind settles, and your headache disappears. You needed the new glasses to see the world more clearly, yet you may not have been aware of that.

Self-assessments are similar. You may not be able to recognize the truth unless something—or someone—points it out to you. For that reason, these assessments are most helpful when conducted with some supervision and guidance. Starting the self-inquiry process is meaningful, yet the greatest outcome will occur with an observer, such as a provider or a loved one, who can reflect on your answers—and even make sure you provide the best ones.

If I asked you, for example, if you are someone who listens well, your response would be based on whether you *believe* you listen well. Unfortunately, the MOW behind your answer may not be true. You see your truth through your own eyes—yet is it really the truth? Only those who spend time with you can truly answer that question.

Importantly, a guide's responses are based upon their beliefs—their MOW—about what makes a good listener. So, it would take many eyes and a lot of observation to give the best answer. Make sense? This is where things can get tricky. If your guide is not balanced with him or herself, their assessment may not be very helpful in the long run. Over the last two decades of speaking and educating clinicians, I have met many physicians. Very often, I found the physician was not internally connected or balanced.

If that is the case, how can they guide you on your imbalances?

I believe we must practice what we preach . . . especially as providers yet also as parents, significant others, caregivers, and friends.

If I ask you if you are a good listener, for me to assess your listening skills, I would only feel comfortable doing so if I understood what it meant to be a good listener. That would take me understanding if I am a good listener too. Since I have spent two decades observing other patients and clients and also spent time working on my listening skills through yoga, breathwork, and meditation, I feel that this is a question I am worthy of assessing. Because I have been too windy and spent more time talking than listening, I became motivated to start working on myself before helping others. During my excessively windy personality days, this nature led to me misinterpreting others, leading to poor understanding at times. From these experiences, I have begun to embrace how to be more connected with my true, balanced self versus my imbalanced stress personality. I now attract things in my life that align more with what I am seeking. This has allowed me to have more harmonious relationships and outcomes, along with connecting more deeply with others.

When Dr. Oz's producer invited me back to discuss the Ayurvedic stress types, I told her that Ayurveda doesn't look at the stress type. The goal of Ayurvedic assessments is to understand your balanced, non-stressed self, known as your prakruti. She insisted that this was what Dr. Oz and the executive team wanted me to discuss.

I thought long and hard about whether I should do the segment and finally decided to do it anyway. I am glad I did. It was one of the most pivotal experiences in my life. I realized what the show and the audience wanted was exactly what my patients needed. It was time for me to evolve the way I assessed patients. I would focus on first determining what aspect of an individual was out of alignment. Then I would recommend techniques to improve that aspect, thereby revealing their true nature.

To spend time in atma vichara, you should clear the imbalance state or personality that has formed to protect you from danger. Your goal is to identify which personality you have taken on, why you have chosen that personality, and clear the programming behind it to clear reptilian brain dominance. Remember we would like to balance the hemispheres of the brain so your prefrontal cortex, which aligns with your joyous and harmonious inner self, comes out of hiding. The reptilian and limbic brains have been hijacking it for too long.

A balanced brain is a whole brain and, thus, it supports whole-body coherence and alignment.

For this reason, I created the stress personality quiz referred to in the introduction.[2] If you haven't already done so, please take this quiz. It will help you determine your stress personality type: imbalanced vata, pitta, or kapha.

Additionally, I utilize the stress personality quiz as another way to assess the guna of your mind. Gunas are considered to be the core dynamic forces of nature, and the predominant guna of the mind allows you to understand how you respond to the world around you. *Guna*, which in Sanskrit implies the "quality or tendency that is present in all living things," is another way of understanding your personality. The three gunas are sattva, rajas, and tamas. Sattva infers a harmonious and calm personality; rajas infers a passionate or driven personality; and tamas infers a lazy or ignorant personality. The quiz gives insight into how your mind is influenced by the force of nature.

Living in a stressful state leads to an imbalanced personality, thus blocking success and happiness in many areas of life. The inauthentic you that results from stress lives in survival mode. Learn to identify with this state and bring it into balance so you can reach inner bliss and harmony.

THIS IS THE STRESS RX

When I was interviewed to join a business fraternity in my first year of college, the kind interviewer gave me a copy of the famous poem about success often attributed to Ralph Waldo Emerson:

To laugh often and much
To win the respect
Of intelligent persons
And the affection of children;
To hear the approbation
Of honest critics;
To appreciate the beauty:
to give of one's self;
To know even one life
Has breathed easier
Because you have lived-
That is to have succeeded.[3]

What defines success for you?

Think about all areas of your life—family, friends, health, career, personal growth, and spirituality. Being successful means being in alignment with your values and goals in all areas of life. If you struggle in one area, it will impact success in other areas. For example, if you have health challenges, your career will be impacted. Emphasizing success in one area may disrupt another area. Focusing on a career may disrupt relationships or family. Determine what success means for you to create balance.

Since discovering what success and balance means for me, the way I work has dramatically changed. Simply working hard did not lead to my definition of success. Rather, it led me to an imbalanced personality that was constantly trying to achieve something. No matter how incredible any of my accomplishments were, I was never really satisfied with them.

Around 2013, when I began transcendental meditation and left the wellness center I was codirecting, life began to shift in a big way. I finally started focusing on my imbalanced self and cleared some deep baggage. I evaluated all areas of my life and reassessed my values and goals in each area. I worked less and worked smarter instead. I experienced greater personal success with friends and family and greater financial success. As my system moved into coherence, inner conflict and my imbalanced state finally dissolved.

I am far from perfect and still have a way to go, yet I am proud of what I have accomplished. I look forward to continuing the journey.

TAKE-HOME POINTS

1. Your ego is your sense of self, and it is often attached to a wide array of external desires to substantiate its identity. This leads to excess DMN activity. Resistance occurs when you are in this attached state.

2. Maya is a state of illusion. You live in this state when you don't see things as they are. This occurs when your ego is imbalanced and you are connected with your false self versus your true self. This leads down a path of life that does not align with your true nature.

3. Attachments pull you out of alignment. Suppose you are attached to your thoughts, beliefs, or even your physical body. The attachment to those factors can prevent you from being present

for external tasks or the needs of others, further unbalancing your ego.

4. A healthy ego represents a healthy sense of self. This reflects resilience and provides clarity along life's path.

5. Eastern medicine incorporates the subtle body—mind, emotions, and breath—into achieving health. True health occurs when you move beyond focusing on the physical body alone. Clearing the blocks, attachments, and programs in your subtle body helps you move into a deeper sense of balance.

6. Assessing your stress personality type by taking the quiz will help you identify your state imbalance and begin the journey to balance your nature.*

SELF-CARE TIME

Take the following ego attachment quiz and then watch the video, "Ego Attachment," to learn about your results.**

1. Which pronoun do you use most often in conversation?

    a. I

    b. Me

    c. You

    d. We

2. How do you feel when another person succeeds (especially if they are in your area of work or interest)?

    a. I get upset as good things often do not happen for me.

    b. I secretly wish it were me, yet do not get very emotional.

    c. I feel nothing, good or bad.

    d. I feel happy for the other person.

---

*   Take the stress personality quiz at www.truptigokanimd.com/stressrxbonus.

**   To watch "Ego Attachment," visit www.truptigokanimd.com/stressrxbonus.

3. Being famous or recognized, accepted, or approved

   a. is very important to me.

   b. is somewhat important to me.

   c. doesn't matter too much to me.

   d. is something I never think about.

4. How many valuables do you possess (nice clothes, shoes, jewelry, and so on)?

   a. Too much, I admit it!

   b. More than most, yet not too much.

   c. An average amount.

   d. Hardly anything, I don't like to have too many things.

5. When my child grew up and left the house (or when I moved from or left my pet, close friend, or family member or they passed)

   a. I was upset for about a week.

   b. I was upset for a month.

   c. I was upset for months.

   d. I never got over it.

6. You find that you must talk to your parents, siblings, and or kids

   a. daily.

   b. every other day.

   c. weekly.

   d. monthly.

7. What role does drama play in your life?

   a. My life is full of this, and I tend to attract it.

   b. I have a good amount, yet it is more with others I spend time with.

   c. I have more than some, yet not an excessive amount.

   d. I do not have drama.

8. When you are out with others, the conversation is

   a. mainly stories you tell about yourself and your life.
   b. often stories about you or your life.
   c. occasionally stories about you or your life.
   d. rarely stories about you or yourself.

9. How do you feel when someone else gets the attention around you?

   a. I feel unhappy and wish the attention were directed to me.
   b. It's OK if it doesn't last very long.
   c. I try to bring the attention back to me as soon as able.
   d. It doesn't bother me who gets the attention.

10. How do you feel about spending time alone?

    a. I avoid it.
    b. I will do it once in a while.
    c. I am pretty comfortable with it.
    d. I love it.

11. I often try things (foods, activities) that are out of my comfort zone or hang out with different types of people.

    a. Never, I have certain things/foods I enjoy doing and people I prefer to be with.
    b. Sometimes, I will try something new or hang out with someone different, yet usually it's with the same group and activities/foods I am comfortable with.
    c. Often, I try new activities, foods, and people.
    d. Always, variety in activities, foods, and friends is what creates enjoyment in my life.

12. I do volunteer work or am involved in charitable organizations

    a. never.

    b. rarely.

    c. regularly.

    d. often.

13. Do you involve yourself in charity for recognition and status or the social aspects of it over the charitable cause at hand?

    a. Yes

    b. No

14. I am open to listening to others' opinions or advice.

    a. Not open.

    b. Guardedly open.

    c. Open.

    d. Very open.

15. How easy is it for you to accept your role in something or apologize for something that has gone wrong?

    a. I do not like to apologize or accept fault.

    b. Mildly doable. It is a big struggle, and others have told me it's something for me to work on, yet others seem to be to blame most of the time.

    c. I am getting better, yet it's hard as I think others tend to be to blame.

    d. It's very easy for me to apologize or accept fault.

16. Do you follow the rules?

    a. No, I tend to do things my way.

    b. Occasionally, yet at times I like to break them.

    c. Often, I think it's important to follow them.

    d. Always.

17. How long does it take you to ask another how they are?

    a. I rarely do it.

    b. I sometimes remember, yet I often forget.

    c. I ask relatively quickly.

    d. I ask right away.

18. How comfortable are you talking about your emotions?

    a. Never do it.

    b. Rarely, and only if pushed.

    c. I often go there.

    d. I am very comfortable.

Tally the number of times you selected each a, b, c, or d.

    a. _____

    b. _____

    c. _____

    d. _____

11

True Health

What does it mean to be healthy? How do you know if you are truly healthy?

I cannot begin to tell you how many patients have come in to see me over the years after struggling with numbness, pain, insomnia, twitching, headaches, and other ailments, only to be told by their doctors that they were healthy. Their labs and physical exams were "normal," and imaging tests showed a perfectly intact brain. They were told to stop worrying, relax more, and with that, symptoms should hopefully improve. It is not a fault of the doctor, yet our system and how we are trained in medical school. We are trained to diagnose and prescribe.

One of my patients had visited a movement disorders specialist for a tremor. After being assured that her exam and imaging were normal, and the tremor too mild for medication, she was sent on her way with instructions to return if her symptoms worsened. That was it. No diagnosis provided.

What type of health care system tells patients to see doctors only when their symptoms worsen? With that attitude so prevalent, I have heard from many patients who self-medicate, resort to Dr. Google for symptom reduction, and avoid seeking medical attention during the earlier stages of any illness or disfunction when attention would do the most good. It may take months or years before a patient sees their doctor. This can lead to progression of the imbalance, which further increases the likelihood of disease.

The Western definition of health shared in the introduction describes health as the state of being free from illness or injury. By now, you're probably wondering if health is to simply be free of illness or injury. You may be told you are healthy because you do not have diabetes, an autoimmune disease, or cancer—disorders discovered through commonly issued tests—but what if you carry extra weight around your midline or have blood sugar issues not yet manifested as diabetes? Simply because you do not have a current diagnosis or condition does not imply you are healthy.

The WHO definition proposed by Dr. Andrija Štampar, a prominent scholar from Croatia, states that "health is a state of complete physical, mental, and social well-being and not merely the absence of disease or infirmity." This definition seems more in alignment with true health and with my discoveries about Ayurveda.

In my early twenties, as I struggled with debilitating sleep issues, I was told I was healthy. Only after spending time in the bookstore and learning about the Ayurvedic perspective on health did I begin to understand how unhealthy I truly was. According to the Ayurvedic definition, health is more than simply being free of illness or injury. It expands to include a strong agni (digestive fire) along with balance of the mind, senses, and soul.

Read that again and ask yourself: am I truly healthy?

After reading the preceding chapters and exploring the more subtle elements of health—including the sense organs and the mind—you may have a better understanding of what it takes to be truly healthy. So, what is missing in the Western approach to health? It is the lack of understanding the subtle energy body—the forgotten body—which needs attention to be healthy in mind, body, and spirit.

SUBTLE BODY AND LIFE FORCE

Subtle is an often-misunderstood word. It does not mean insignificant. Simply because something is subtle does not imply it lacks power. The subtle body is not readily apparent to the naked eye, yet it is ever-present, influencing the physical body. The subtle body includes senses, life force energy, emotions, thoughts, and the way our experiences and energy flow.

Your senses are part of your subtle, often forgotten body. Are you in touch with each of your five senses: taste, touch, smell, sound, and sight? How do you engage with them each day? What foods do you expose yourself to—processed fare or nutrition provided by nature? How about smells? Do you engage your sense of smell—like stopping to smell the roses—or are you always in a rush, not making time to experience nature or the power of scent? How about sights and sounds? Which types of music or television balance you? Maybe you have some tunes that spark happiness or fond memories, others that help you focus or concentrate, and still other that relax you. Do you take the time to connect with these sounds? Same with your sight. What programs do you watch? Are they violent or soothing? Stimulating or relaxing? If you pay attention, you'll see how your emotional state connects with the reactions of your subtle body, and you will learn to honor both.

Life force is known as prana in Ayurveda or chi in Chinese medicine. It's the energy that allows humans to shine, similar to the electricity lighting a bulb. Although you cannot see the energy, you can see its impact. And sometimes, it's palpable. When someone walks into the room, depending upon your sensitivity, you can usually feel whether their energy is positive or negative.

Can you connect with your own energy? You probably notice when you feel off or unconnected to your most blissful self. Remember the anandamaya kosha? This is the bliss layer or sheath of the subtle body. If you cannot connect with your bliss, the subtle body's outer layers—such as the mind or body—are holding you back.

Your life force influences your thoughts and emotions and vice versa. If you are stuck in a negative thinking pattern, you feel it energetically. The weight of negativity holds you back in every area of life, which only fuels the problem. A more upbeat thinking pattern increases your energy, allowing you to be more receptive, open, and giving in your relationships and family connections.

Emotional connection is often the most challenging area for many people. Emotions are often referred to as "energy in motion." Sorrow, anger, frustration, guilt, regret, shame, or loneliness influence the deepest level of being. If emotions aren't dealt with daily, they may get trapped in the subtle body, leading to physical issues over time. Studies now show that emotions lead to physical body sensations. Difficult emotions such as anxiety and anger most commonly impact the chest area, correlating with changes in heart rate and breathing.[1]

Connecting with physical sensations and recognizing the emotions attached to them allow us to tap into the subtle emotional body. Often our thinking brain and outwardly focused lifestyle prevent us from connecting with these emotional sensations. Most people do not spend enough time in silence to notice how emotions show up physically, either because they have not allowed the time or they tried and were unable to sit for long. Sitting in silence is particularly challenging for those immersed in the individualistic Western society, which focuses on productivity, materialism, and achievement. Society does not encourage "doing nothing."

Eventually, when sensations are dismissed rather than processed over a period of time, they manifest in the subtle body. Dr. Hamer, a German medical doctor, was able to discover a precise correlation between physical symptoms, the brain, and unexpected emotional distress. He called them "conflict shocks." Resolving the emotional conflict led to an improvement in physical symptoms.[2].

This is one of the key areas Western practitioners are not trained to address. Emotions are held in the nervous system if they are not allowed to be processed and cleared. One of the first books I read on this subject, back in 1993, was written by Dr. Bernie Siegel, an assistant clinical professor of general and pediatric surgery at Yale. As a surgeon who focused on removing cancerous masses from the body, he felt unfulfilled and began exploring a deeper understanding of why patients developed cancer in the first place. He began to study how the suppression or release of emotions was linked to cancer development or remission.

In his book *Love, Medicine & Miracles*, Dr. Siegel stated, "Dramatic remissions could occur if patients simply gave up their emotional repression, without chemotherapy or radiation." He went on to say that Mogens Jensen of the Yale psychology department found that, among those with breast cancer, "defensive repressors" die faster than those with a more realistic outlook. A "defensive repressor" is an individual who says, "I am fine," for example, when struggling with something traumatic, such as cancer.[3] Emotions and the lack of connection to them have been proven to have an impact on disease.

We know that the ENS, the nervous system within the gut, is a peripheral extension of the limbic, feeling brain. It contains 200 to 600 million neurons, more neurons than the spinal cord. And it's where the proverbial butterflies appear when you are about to speak in front of a crowd or take a test.

Each emotion carries a vibrational energy. Thus, the array of emotions you display is directly linked to your energy state, your life force. Holding onto emotions like anger, resentment, and frustration affects the energy body. If an uncomfortable emotion is *repressed*, it remains in your subconscious mind, without conscious awareness. It is hidden rather than processed, because it's too painful to approach. *Suppressed* emotions, on the other hand, are consciously hidden because a choice was made to avoid dealing with them. This may happen when the tools for dealing with them, or even the capacity to handle them, is not available.

Whether repressed or suppressed, difficult emotions get stuck in your subtle body. Clearing these emotions—dealing with them— allows the energy state to improve, moving into a higher vibration, which is linked to joy, gratitude, inspiration, and vibrancy.

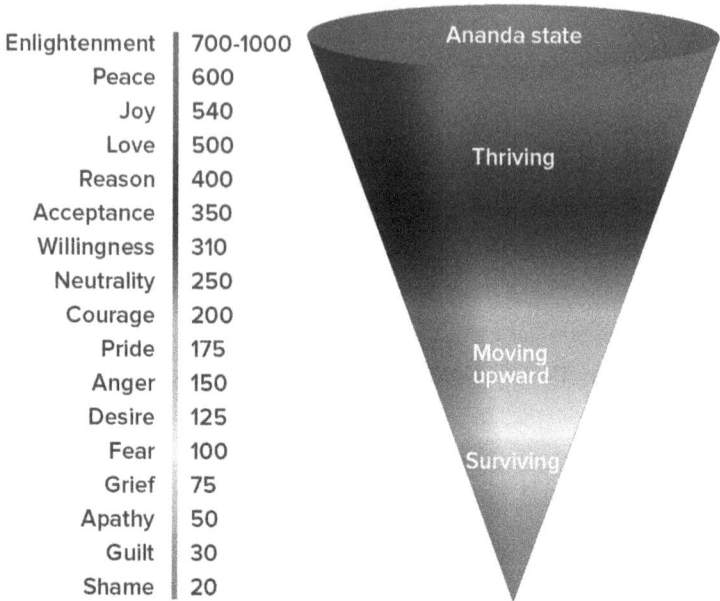

Enlightenment	700-1000	Ananda state
Peace	600	
Joy	540	
Love	500	Thriving
Reason	400	
Acceptance	350	
Willingness	310	
Neutrality	250	
Courage	200	
Pride	175	
Anger	150	Moving upward
Desire	125	
Fear	100	
Grief	75	Surviving
Apathy	50	
Guilt	30	
Shame	20	

Copyright@2021TruptiGokanIMD

In the image in figure 11.1, you can see how emotions are linked to certain vibrational energy levels. This is based on one of the most profound books I have read, *Power vs. Force* by Sir David Hawkins, MD, PhD.[4] I found this book in a quaint café outside of Maharishi University, where I had just given a talk on menstrual migraines. I sought more wisdom from ancient thinkers and found this brilliant book discussing how to operate from a sense of power and influence rather than force.

Powerful, virtuous leaders such as Mahatma Gandhi or Martin Luther King Jr. use thinking and philosophy to inspire change. Forceful leaders like Hitler or Idi Amin use intimidation and fear to coerce change. The vibrational tendency, or energy, behind those leaders reflects their life force. Those who inspire have a higher, positive life force. Those who must coerce have a lower, negative vibration.

Think of someone you know who has a high-vibe personality. What is their nature and personality? Are they angry and anxious or inspiring and joyful to be around? Based on muscle testing, Dr. Hawkins could map out an individual's energetic patterns and which specific emotions their system was holding onto.

Each of us holds onto emotions, even if we aren't aware of them. The goal is to clear the stuck energies linked to the emotions that are not serving you, thus allowing you to move toward a higher vibration.

Our discussion of ego attachments revealed that being attached to your physical body may be linked to a deep feeling of shame. You may obsess about your weight, including your food and workouts, and obsess over overlooking "perfect," as it helps mitigate your feeling of shame. Understanding this attachment and then clearing the emotion underneath it will allow you to release the heavy negative emotional energy surrounding your body image. Then, you move to a higher vibe state, where you can perform at your optimal level in mind, body, and spirit.

Incredibly, as you clear your imbalanced emotions and improve your vibrational energy, you naturally become healthier and happier, thus shedding those pounds you so desperately wanted to lose in the first place.

Hawkins's book shifted me tremendously. I was finally able to understand the energy body of Ayurveda and the connection between our emotional patterns and behavior styles.

To find true health, you must clear lower emotions of shame, guilt, grief, fear, desire, and anger and move toward higher emotions, such as joy and gratitude, which are linked to higher energy or life force. These lower emotions are connected to your attachments. Thus, as you work on clearing your attachments, you naturally move up into a higher vibrational state.

This is the essence of balancing your subtle body.

Atma vichara, the soul analysis discussed in chapter 10, occurs when you find your true self. This sense of knowing extends beyond the thinking mind (the manas). It is the pure essence of who you are without your attachments, a knowing that empowers you to truly live. Your ego is healthy and balanced. You feel whole, entirely as you are. You do not depend on others or derive happiness from attachments. Material items seem less important when feeling happy or fulfilled. With the ability to feel the high vibrations of bliss on your own, you naturally attract equally high vibrational situations and individuals in your life.

There is no duality in this state. There is no *you versus me*; no *you versus them*. Your imbalance or false ego has dissolved into a state of balanced ego and sense of self. You know you are part of the energy in all, in the universe. You feel connected and aligned with the world around you. When you live a life aligned with this true self, your life becomes incredible. You attain health, peace, and prosperity quickly and effortlessly. You find authentic happiness.

BRAIN HEALTH EXPANDED

As I embraced these teachings about the subtle body and life force energy in my practice, I began to expand on the definition of brain health. My moods, along with my health, were at the best place they had been in years. I wanted nothing more than to share the steps needed to arrive at this state with others. But I needed more than the conventional model to get there.

In traditional neurology, we are trained to believe two main operating systems regulate us: the CNS—the brain in your head, along with the spinal cord—and the PNS, the nerves that branch from your CNS to your body. The PNS includes the autonomic nervous system (ANS). Generally, the ANS is believed to have two parts, the sympathetic and parasympathetic divisions, which regulate your fight or flight or rest and digest states, among other things. Yet researchers such as Dr. Gershon, who wrote the book *The Second Brain*, believe that the enteric nervous system, ENS, described above, is the third part of the ANS.[5] The reason is, with 200 to 600 million neurons in the gut, the ENS is a complex system that can function without intervention from the CNS. It can operate on its own. This, along with his research revealing the multitude of neurotransmitters produced in the ENS, led to his belief that the ENS should have its division and importance.

ANS → SNS, PNS, & ENS

This system, I began to realize, was one of the missing pieces in conquering health challenges. After studying the patients who were able to transform their health, I realized that their recovery could be explained in a three brain model incorporating more aspects of our being than traditionally taught in medical school and residency.

THE THREE BRAINS

That discovery led me to create the Three Brain Optimization Program. This model evaluates the *thinking* brain, the *feeling* brain, and the *doing* brain and assesses the health of each. Most of us will have some imbalance in each brain, yet one brain may dominate the imbalance. If that's the case, we must pay attention to it first.

The easiest way to conceptualize "brain" is to view it as the part of us that works as a system to control our human experience. This three brain model has given me a clear framework I can use to work with patients and clients to achieve stress reduction, thereby improving happiness in life and resulting in more abundant health.

The First Brain

The first brain, the CNS, represents the thinking brain. This is the brain that allows the formation of thoughts and beliefs. It holds a person's programming. The CNS represents an individual's MOW, as discussed in chapter 4. The MOW is created from childhood experiences, which are influenced by socioeconomic status, religion, culture, living environment, parental influences, and so on. Each individual has a unique MOW and first brain pattern, based not only on how they were raised but also on how much they absorbed from their environment, combined with their unique interpretation of the events.

For example, someone who grew up in a quiet and serene countryside may believe that working in a big city would be distracting and anxiety-provoking. Someone raised in the city may believe that working there provides opportunity for creativity and enhances productivity. These perspectives are based on the unique programs of the individual and how they interpreted their experiences. No right or wrong, just different models. Even twins brought up by the very same parents can develop different perspectives on their lives due to their individual interpretations of experiences with their family, friends, and society.

The goal is to evaluate if your first brain MOW is giving you harmony or creating distress.

The Second Brain

The second brain, the ENS, is the feeling brain. This is the brain that picks up on emotions and connects to the intuitive center. For many people, including me, expressing emotions was not encouraged during early life. I remember crying as I told a relative about a challenge in middle school at a family gathering. This close family member told me I shouldn't cry; I shouldn't be so sensitive about it. When a child is advised not to cry or be angry, they are receiving instructions to suppress emotions instead of expressing them. Expressing feelings is key to a healthy ENS.

Another way to get into your emotional body is by honoring your natural circadian rhythms, such as setting mealtimes and bedtime routines. The more you get aligned with your natural rhythm of cortisol and natural urges to eat, sleep, and rest, you naturally become more connected with your emotional self. Ignoring your circadian rhythms traps energy in your body or leads to emotional dysregulation, resulting in chronic neck pain, back pain, digestive issues, immune imbalances, and more. In two decades of practice, I have seen this situation impact patients many times over. Thus, acknowledging the health of this area is key to balancing your system and reaching optimal well-being.

The Third Brain

The third brain, the doing brain, is your gut microbiome. It consists of the 100 trillion bacteria, viruses, and organisms that lie within your digestive system. These microbiota are responsible for fermenting proteins and carbohydrates, creating metabolic by-products to help repair and strengthen the gut and immune system, absorb nutrients, and create neurotransmitters and vitamins. If these organisms are not in alignment, your unique physiology and environment imbalance occurs at this level. You may not produce essential fatty acids, such as butyrate, which strengthen the membrane of the gut and stabilize the brain. As a result, neurotransmitter production suffers. Because 70 percent of your immune function resides in your gut, your immune system weakens. These are just a few of the possible challenges. To create a healthy third brain, the microbiome must undergo specific testing. The diet must consist of foods and spices that nourish microbiota. Even eating at the right time of the day can influence microbiome health.

Three Brain Interaction

This is both a top-down and bottom-up approach where you can throw your second brain and third brain off-balance with negative, unproductive thoughts in the first brain. A first brain imbalance prevents you from feeling and connecting with your emotions.

Perfectionism and people-pleasing commonly imbalances the first brain, and it's something I'm familiar with. Thankfully, I now have the awareness and tools to help reduce idealistic thoughts, which lead to behaviors that further imbalance me. When stuck in thought, we often spin into actions that don't serve us (fight or flight state) or immobilize us (freeze state). Each of these states leads to an adrenal imbalance, eventually creating imbalance in second and third brain function.

If I am too busy doing and performing, I will not allow myself to feel or process what is underneath the imbalanced action. I may aim for perfection because I do not feel worthy to obtain my goal. This further impairs the microbiome, thus leading to a top-down imbalance.

How does that happen? When under stress, the body naturally diverts blood flow from the gut to the skeletal muscles in preparation to escape danger. Who has time to sit and eat a sandwich when a bear is chasing you? Chronic stress can lead to digestive impairments. Studies show that stress leads to a reduction in microbiome lactobacilli along with an increase in pathogenic (unhealthy) bacteria strains such as pseudomonas and *E. coli*.[6]

Most neurological disorders are linked to pathogens in the gut. The presence of these pathogens may lead to an impairment of gut motility by reducing tight junction proteins, the building blocks of the gut barrier. Reduction of tight junction proteins may cause a leaky gut, also known as increased intestinal permeability.[7] A leaky gut leads to a release of lipopolysaccharide (LPS), a cellular wall component of certain bacteria, into the bloodstream. This elevates inflammatory cytokines, which cause inflammation throughout the body.

Similarly, suppose gut bacteria are imbalanced with high levels of pathogenic bacteria or a low diversity of healthy bugs. That can cause depression or anxiety and perpetuate negative thoughts. Researchers have found specific types of bacteria present in families with depression.[8] In addition, some bacteria may impact the ability to perceive stress, leading to a reduction in cortisol production.[9] Other studies reveal that timid mice became bold and adventurous after shifting their

microbiome. They also shifted their production of brain-derived neu-
rotrophic factor (BDNF), which is a protein linked to new neuronal
sprouting and improvement in brain function, especially in the hippocampus.[10] This is the bottom-up way in which we can feel out of
alignment with a higher risk of mood disorders and impaired stress
responses.

Who is in control? Your first, second, or third brain?

The jury is out, yet science shows there is more conversation from
the gut to the brain than the brain to the gut. Fascinating! Parkinson's
disease is one of the most disabling neurodegenerative diseases known
to humankind. An abundance of emerging research links the mind-
gut-brain interaction to this disease. It is believed that the first symptoms patients have are anxiety and constipation. These may occur as
early as twenty years before the tremors or slow movement associated
with Parkinson's make an appearance.[11] Another study hypothesized
that there are two subtypes of Parkinson's. One is brain-first (top-
down) and the other is body-first (bottom-up). In the brain-first sub-
type, alpha-synuclein arises in the brain and spreads to the peripheral
ANS. In the body-first (bottom-up) type, the pathology originates in
the ENS and spreads to the brain.[12]

I used to believe the brain in our heads was in charge, yet now,
after years of practice, I am not quite sure who is really in charge.

SPIRITUALITY AND HEALTH

A key aspect of true health is being connected to your spiritual self. So,
what does it mean to be spiritual? To some, spirituality means knowing
that there is an inner spirit or soul that is always guiding you. This soul
was present at birth and is with you until you leave this earth.

This idea often extends to include the connection of this spirit or
soul with a higher energy source. This energy source may be derived
from the planets. It may have no form yet be considered a higher power.

Those who are religious may believe that this higher power takes the form of a particular god or figure and follows a set of scriptures or beliefs. Often associated with religion, spirituality is the belief in something bigger than yourself and knowing that this source supports your soul as you journey through life. That support may come in the way of enhanced intuition or an inner knowing about a given situation or decision. It may appear as guidance or direction when you are feeling lost. The guidance may help you move forward.

For example, when our children were young and we were in the midst of a home search, we lived in a rental townhome. There was nothing on the market in the area we wished to live. After one typical Sunday morning yoga class and meditation, I walked down a specific street in the adjacent neighborhood. I loved the feel of the street and that part of town. I felt a calling to that area. *I would love it if one of these houses went on the market,* I thought. After arriving home, I went to the neighborhood listserv and asked if anyone was planning on selling. Within an hour, a response came from a woman whose house was on that very same street. She planned to put her home on the market in two months, yet said she would show it to me if I were interested. Remember, nothing was available at that time. We had been searching for nine months! Yet, on this specific day, I had clarity about exactly where I wanted to be.

As they say, *ask and you shall receive.* We ended up signing a contract for that house without it ever being in the market. It may seem like a coincidence, yet situations like these have happened to me quite a few times in my life.

The key to finding what you want or need is being clear about what you want and desiring it for the highest intentions. To me, this is an example of divine intervention. If it is meant to be, being spiritual or religious allows answers to show up in your life with the assistance of something greater than yourself.

In another situation, I was slotted to do a segment on national TV in New York City about a twenty-one-day turmeric tonic challenge.

We had lost my husband's first cousin the week the show was to air. With my mind so distraught after this loss, I called the producer to tell her I didn't think I was capable of doing the show. Dressing up, getting hair and makeup done, and being on camera with all the media attention, seemed inappropriate when mourning a loss. The producer convinced me to do it anyway. They had a group of audience members who completed the challenge, and I was the only one versed in the material. It would be hard to cancel.

I felt torn, yet I decided to be open to what would come.

As I made my way to the airport, I heard that flights were being canceled due to weather on the East Coast. I felt that maybe it was meant to be that I wouldn't be doing the show after all. After checking in for my flight and realizing the earlier flight was canceled, the airline attendant said she'd put me down on the standby list for the flight leaving later that night . . . in case my flight was canceled. I sat down and opened *The Universe Has Your Back* by Gabby Bernstein.[13] As I waited for my flight to board, I immersed myself in this book. I looked up what seemed like hours later to find out my flight was canceled. I decided to wait and hear what happened to the following flight. Remarkably, the next flight was cleared to fly, and they called one—and only one—standby passenger to board the flight. It was me. I was stunned. As I went to board, I passed at least a hundred disgruntled faces—all the other standby passengers. I had no special status, yet I somehow made it on. Although this was surprising for me, what happened next was somewhat incomprehensible.

After landing in New York, I made my way to the same hotel I stayed in the last time I came for the show. I visualized doing morning yoga, then felt a touch of despair knowing how small the hotel room would be. Yet, with no conversation, the hotel attendant told me she was going to put me in a nice room. I thanked her and made my way up to the eleventh floor, where I realized she had moved me to the penthouse unit! It made no sense. Again, I had zero status. I hadn't even told her why I was in New York. I had an entire living room area with two walls of windows. Plenty of space to do yoga.

I began to question how things had lined up for me to be on the show. I kept reading *The Universe Has Your Back,* believing that if I were meant to be there, the universe would let me know. The following day, I made my way to the studio. Typically, in the green room area (the space where guests prep before the show), I leave my door open to meet the other guests filming that day. I have met many celebrities and other fascinating individuals that way. In the past, I would watch the segment before mine and then make my way to the stage. This time, I told the producer to call me only when it was time to go on. I didn't watch the show. In my grief, I kept the door closed and meditated.

I completed my segment, grateful I could serve the audience and viewers with Ayurvedic remedies to improve mental and physical health. I felt that this message was important to share and that is why it all aligned for me to be there. As I left the studio after the recording, I told my producer to read *The Universe Has Your Back.* I shared how uncanny it was that I made the flight and was upgraded to the penthouse suite. I felt as though I was being taken care of by some greater power during this difficult time. I felt safe and protected, as the book describes.

She told me she would indeed buy the book and read it. As I made my way back to the green room, I noticed someone walking in front of me with beautiful blonde hair. She looked angelic—and familiar. I paused. *It couldn't be.*

I walked up to the woman and tapped her shoulder. As she turned around, I was stunned.

I said, "Hi . . . Are you Gabby Bernstein?"

She smiled and said yes. I shared my experience and how her book was quite helpful for me during this difficult time. She told me she was grateful that it served me. It turned out that her room was directly across the hall from mine. I called my producer in shock, and she told me she was working on my segment and another, thus had no idea who else was filming that day. She was equally surprised, to say the least.

To make the story even more interesting, when the segment aired a month later, guess who was on right before me? Yes, Gabby Bernstein. Her segment was a twenty-one-day sugar-elimination challenge.

I was stunned yet felt something besides my own free will allowed this magical sequence of events and connection to happen. Some call these a series of God-winks: gentle reminders that something greater than us helps us along this journey of life. After a troubling week of losing someone I loved, I felt the universe had let me know it was right to go on the show and share my work with others. I felt at peace with it all, just what I was hoping for.

You may think these situations are merely coincidental, yet I believe I was in alignment with a higher power which allowed these outcomes to manifest. We are each entitled to our own belief system. I am not here to convince anyone of my belief system. I am simply here to share my journey and thoughts, allowing you all to assess this in a way that makes sense for you. It's a very personal decision.

I do not have proof, just a sense of knowing that something more intelligent than us created this universe and the human species. Otherwise, how is it that our hearts beat, we release digestive enzymes, we coordinate our bodies to think and move, and most of it without our conscious awareness? We, as humans, are not intelligent enough to do this. How is the universe so perfectly organized to provide Mother Earth with what is needed for life, plants, and species to thrive?

Visiting ancient ruins, such as during our hike up to Machu Picchu, certain feats are inexplicable—like structures that seem impossible to create with human intervention alone. How did they come to be?

The more I tune into my inner knowing and ask the universe for support, the more readily things move into alignment in my life.

You may not be sure how all this is all links to health. The subtle body, holding your thoughts, emotions, senses, and spirituality, and its impact on your well-being may seem foreign and intangible. I appreciate this; in these modern times, we have not been trained to think of health in this more holistic way.

It is fascinating to review research about how being spiritual or religious affects your health. Studies reveal that less spiritual adolescents
are more likely to use substances such as alcohol or tobacco. We know
the use of these substances is linked to both physical and mental health
issues.[14] Those with a more spiritual perspective on life have improved
psychological well-being and a reduction in stress, both of which contribute to improved health.[15] Further research shows that individuals
who attend religious services have a decrease in inflammatory cytokines such as IL-6, along with enhanced longevity.[16]

Whether you choose to be spiritual or participate in religious services is entirely up to you. I personally find this research fascinating
and believe if we discover more tools to improve our health and longevity, why not consider them?

TAKE-HOME POINTS

1. The modern definition of health is missing the aspect of the subtle body. The soul, sense organs, and mind are not routinely part
   of the Western definition of health yet are of high importance in
   the Eastern definition.

2. Your energy, or life force or prana, is important to evaluate as
   it is linked to your sense of well-being. Your energy is linked to
   your vibrational state.

3. Your lower vibrational emotions, which are connected to your
   attachments, must be cleared so you can move to a higher vibrational state and live in alignment with your most optimal,
   balanced self.

4. Your number one goal is to clear out the baggage inherited from
   early life programs and trauma so that you may function at your
   highest potential. This is the high-vibe state that allows you to
   feel joyful, grateful, inspired, and vibrant.

5. The three brain approach to health encompasses your first brain (your CNS), your second brain (your ENS), and your third brain (your microbiome). Each plays a role in a top-down and bottom-up way to keep you aligned and optimal. If one brain is out of alignment, it can influence the health of the other brains.

6. Spirituality is very personal. The basic premise involves believing that we have a soul, or spirit, within us. A higher force may guide this soul to support and help direct individuals in life's journey.

7. Studies have demonstrated that practicing religion and/or being spiritual may lead to an improvement in disease and increased longevity.

ACTION STEPS

If you have taken the stress personality quiz, it would be a good time to evaluate the results and even retake it.* To achieve success, spend some time evaluating your stress personality quiz results. Think about why your results are windy, fiery, or earthy.

Circle your results here:

Windy   Fiery   Earthy

Now ask yourself, what led to this state?

With the results of your stress personality in mind, the three brain quiz** will give you a breakdown of the alignment or misalignment in each of your brains.

It took me decades to develop this approach. Once you start applying it to your health, you will see how understanding the health of each brain can help you figure out whether you have true health. If you don't, then you can begin to explore what you need to improve your

---

*   To access the stress personality quiz, visit www.truptigokanimd.com/stressrxbonus.

**   To access the three brain quiz, visit www.truptigokanimd.com/stressrxbonus.

health and avoid or lessen the burden of disease.

Take the Three Brain Quiz*** to help you assess your subtle, forgotten body and understand which aspects of it are requesting the most attention and healing.

Report your results here:

Brain One: _____
Brain Two: _____
Brain Three: _____

Journal any thoughts you have about the quiz results.

Why do you believe you have these results, based on what you have learned?

***   To access the three brain quiz, visit www.truptigokanimd.com/stressrxbonus.

12

Your Body Is Your Messenger

Julie was a vibrant young lady. Consistently coming into my clinic with a smile on her face, she quickly became one of my favorite patients. But one day, she seemed different. She was visibly upset. As she sat on the examination table, she held onto her right shoulder and told me she was struggling. Her migraine hadn't resolved, and she was experiencing severe, daily neck pain. The medications simply did not help. I offered to give her trigger point injections, natural agents that often helped break the cycle of pain. As I prepped her for the injections, I couldn't help but notice the Latin words tattooed on her shoulders: *perfer et obdura; dolor hic tibi proderit olim.*

I asked her the meaning behind the words.

"Be patient and tough; someday this pain will be useful to you," she said, tearing up.

I grabbed her hand and slowly nodded. I felt her pain at that moment. I felt what she was going through. I focused my energy on getting her better and held back tears as I began the injections.

Julie's tattoo, a powerful quote by the famous Roman poet Ovid, caught me off guard. Julie was one of the most resilient patients I knew. She struggled with near-daily pain yet managed to work long hours and study in a graduate program. Somehow, she always seemed to stay upbeat. When she shared the meaning of her tattoo, I felt something different. Her body was telling her something, and we were not listening to the message.

ARE YOU LISTENING?

The physical body is so beautifully designed that if you take care of it, it allows you to operate at your highest level. Eating high-quality foods, surrounding yourself with positive people, and listening to uplifting music make your body feel better. Overtax your body and push beyond your limits, however, and your body will let you know. The pain that occurs in your right knee every time you run or the migraine that comes on when you have your menstrual cycle or during a full moon are messages. Your body is telling you to shift the way you exercise or how you live.

One patient called our office for a refill of triptan, a migraine medication, while she was running errands before a workout class. During her previous visit, I advised her against doing that specific type of workout. I believed it aggravated the migraines she had been experiencing about three times per week. She disregarded my advice and planned to go anyway.

When the instructor did not show up for class—the first time this had happened in two years—my patient decided that maybe the universe was giving her a sign. She stopped her classes for one week—and she did not get a migraine for the entire week. It was the first time in months that she remained pain-free for that long.

On her next visit, she told me the story, laughed, and said, "I guess I should have followed the doctor's advice!"

As I stated previously, my role is not to fix anyone but to guide and educate them so they can be their own healer. Trust that you hold the answers within, that listening to your body will guide you toward the best next step in life. If that leads you to restorative yoga instead of a hot yoga, so be it. The body is always sending messages—not only for you to *hear* the message but to *respond* to it and honor it with a shift in action or behavior.

I'll ask again: are you listening to your body's messages?

THE BODY HOLDS ON

As you know from our previous discussions, the body holds onto stored memories, emotions, and trauma from the past, all of which can impact it physically. Suppose you repress anger. According to Dr. Vasant Lad, one of the most esteemed practitioners and educators of Ayurvedic medicine, that anger can change the flora of your gallbladder, small intestine, and bile duct.[1]

Imagine that. Stored anger can shift your gut flora!

An imbalance in your energy state—when you become too windy, fiery, or earthy—creates emotional and physical symptoms. (See the Dosha Types on page 19 and 20.) Remember Julie, with the severe neck pain and headaches? In her scenario, multitasking at work and school led to a buildup of vata (windy) energy. Vata energy regulates the movement of downward flow. Unfortunately, Julie became constipated (a freeze state) during this time. She was only having a bowel movement every other day. Since the vata energy could not be released from the body, which happens with regular daily elimination, the excess energy moved upward and found its place in her neck.

Neck pain is one of the most common presentations of a vata or windy excess. Imagine going into a freeze state when you perceive danger. Your body becomes small as you tuck yourself in (similar to being in a fetal position), and your neck tightens as you drop your head forward, attempting to hide from danger. In the freeze state, muscles contract, including the colon, and that tightening results in constipation. The colon spasms due to an energetic shift at the gut level.

The solution is not taking more laxatives (which Julie's primary care doctor recommended) but to work on reducing your vata lifestyle. Not easy, yet if that energy isn't released, it accumulates in the body. Eventually, it will show up through more symptoms. If Julie's state were to continue, the vata energy would move into her mind, creating a restless, distracted, anxious, and unfocused mind.

Increased symptoms are a stronger message from the universe encouraging you to stop your windy, fiery, or earthy way of being. Whenever symptoms arise, pause and reflect on why they are happening. In this state, you have an opportunity to reflect on how to shift your life and physiology and take action. If the appropriate shifts are made, the energy body will move back into balance, thus reducing your symptoms. This is the message your body wants you to hear.

WINDY

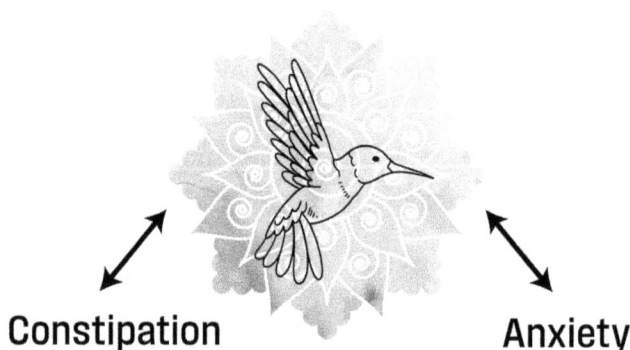

Constipation   Anxiety

SPEND TIME PAYING ATTENTION

To assess your body's energy accumulation and whether it is holding onto the emotions of the past, connect with your physical body. Spend time becoming aware of all its parts and sensations.

Do you wake up with a slight ache in your hip or elsewhere in your body?

Do you develop neck tightness or a headache when having an intense conversation, late at night, or working on the computer?

Explore your aches and pains and the circumstances surrounding them. (You'll find some suggestions for how to do that in the action steps at the end of this chapter.)

This process takes time. Exercises that slow you down, such as yoga or tai chi, improve sensitivity to the physical sensations within your body. Eventually, you will recognize points of tension, the areas where your body holds excess energy. And remember, no matter how far advanced your state of disconnect may be, you can always reengage with yourself. Start listening and interrupt or begin to repair disease development. It is never too late. Never.

Poet Nayyirah Waheed beautifully describes this process: "And I said to my body softly. 'I want to be your friend.' It took a long breath and replied, 'I have been waiting my whole life for this.'"[2]

Read Waheed's words aloud and see how they make you feel. And then ask yourself why you stopped listening to your body. Have you become angry at your symptoms or disease? Are you angry at yourself for not being healthy? No worries, as now is your time to start listening.

The battle with self is common among those who suffer from chronic symptoms or diseases. Repressed emotions often relate to societal expectations. If, for example, you felt shame or guilt when you were younger, you may not have felt safe enough to share it. If that's the case, did your parents, caregivers, sibling, or teachers ever tell you NOT to share your feelings, thoughts, or emotions?

FROM SYMPATHY TO EMPATHY AND COMPASSION

Sympathy, empathy, and compassion all deal with emotional responses to other people—but they each have different implications.

Sympathy is a pity-based response that typically results when feeling sorry for someone without making any attempt to understand what they are going through. Responding with sympathy creates distance. It may make the giver feel better, but it does nothing to help the receiver. A sympathetic response is more about the giver than the receiver.

Empathy, on the other hand, is more about the receiver than the giver. Empathy occurs when we sense another's emotion and are able to imagine what they may be thinking or how they may be feeling. In Sanskrit, this is known as *bhava*, which embodies tenderness and love. According to Brené Brown, one of the world's experts on vulnerability, empathy fuels connection while sympathy drives disconnection. This suggests we cannot begin to be truly vulnerable without empathy for one another.

It is important to note that if one struggles with negative emotions themselves, empathy can be difficult to practice. Becoming vulnerable enough to connect in that way could put you at risk of absorbing another person's emotions or energy. This can be taxing, particularly for highly sensitive persons. Absorbing negativity from another person may cause an energy imbalance and corresponding symptoms, which is not the desired outcome.

Daniel Goleman, renowned psychologist and the author of the bestselling book *Emotional Intelligence: Why It Can Matter More Than IQ*, encourages people to tune into their own emotions and those of others.[3] In his many writings and lectures, he frequently states that empathy requires perspective-taking. It allows you to see the situation from another's MOW instead of solely from your own. This way, you can slide into the other person's shoes to understand what they are struggling with. Doing this well requires releasing any judgment you may have about the person and their situation, acknowledging their emotions, and letting them know you can appreciate what they are feeling.

If extended thoughtfully, empathy allows one person to feel with another, to share their joy and successes along with challenges and struggles. Have you ever experienced a win, something amazing that happened in your life, and it felt like no one else noticed? You were likely seeking empathy and compassion during that time.

Those who have empathy are more likely to develop compassion, which means "to suffer together." Compassion opens us to another individual's struggle at a deeper level and inspires us not just to acknowledge their situation but to help them through it. Compassion reflects the deepest emotional connection possible through vulnerability.

Compassion forms the core of the human experience. Recognizing another person's struggle and helping them get through it—regardless of who they are or how they view the world—is the essence of life.

Showing compassion should be easy enough to do, right?

Then why are so many people challenged with being compassionate?

Too many people allow their fear of vulnerability to hold them back from offering more than sympathy. Move toward compassion by showing empathy for yourself. Recognize and respect your boundaries and what you can handle. Practice empathy with others by connecting with the part of yourself that understands what others are experiencing. If someone is grieving over a loss, connect with your own experiences of loss so that you may feel sorrow along with them.

Empathy was certainly not taught in medical school, resulting in many physicians with poor bedside manners. This is no fault of theirs, simply a fault of their training. During my training, my attending physician suggested either you have it, or you don't. That simply isn't true. I believe empathy can be taught through active listening, and it should be part of the medical school curriculum.

A provider's ability to demonstrate empathy is crucial for developing a trusting relationship with patients. This requires some amount of vulnerability from the provider. For providers who have not developed a connection with their emotional body (a second brain connection), becoming vulnerable and thus empathic is difficult. The beauty is that this can be developed over time if there is a desire to do so.

I mentioned tearing up when my patient Julie told me the meaning of her tattooed quote. I'm curious if you thought that was appropriate for me to do. From my perspective, the ability to connect on an empathic level has genuinely helped me serve patients and clients. Some of my own learning came during my struggle with insomnia. I had to learn to be empathic with myself.

SHARE YOUR EXPERIENCE

When I began struggling with insomnia, I held the story within for the first month, optimistically hoping it would end. When symptoms grew pervasive, affecting my energy and motivation during the day, I began to share with others, hoping for support and guidance.

I spoke openly about it with a medical school friend while we sat in a café. As I revealed my struggles, Jennifer (pseudonym) kept saying how sorry she felt for me. When I mentioned previously sharing my challenge with another friend, Elizabeth (pseudonym), Jennifer encouraged me to keep my struggle quiet. She was concerned that Elizabeth, who had failed to get into medical school, would question my contemplation about leaving and might even share my challenges with our community. People might start talking.

This is a classic example of *schadenfreude*—a German term for gleaning pleasure or satisfaction from another person's misfortune. Supposedly, Jennifer was protecting me from others who secretly wished I would quit. How much of this was true, I didn't know. While I appreciated her efforts to keep me safe from criticism or judgment, it only made my situation worse. The conversation itself left me feeling uneasy and with a panging sense of shame—quite the opposite of what I needed at that time. I craved understanding from others and their encouragement that I would get better, not advice to keep quiet.

Although I did not know it at the time, my subtle body was speaking through my health challenges. It wanted me to speak confidently and openly about my situation to garner the support, love, and tools I needed to move forward. Although that was not the feedback I received, I was, thankfully, surrounded by plenty of spiritual textbooks to guide my path and keep me positive and hopeful. Ayurveda taught me that we were never intended to go it alone—contrary to the social conditioning common among many North Americans. The authors of these books became my support system. They gave me confidence that I wasn't alone on this journey and that I would get through it.

You may also find you do not have a safe space in which to reveal your deepest feelings and truths. Maybe you fear criticism, judgment, or shame. This reasoning keeps most people stuck in their comfort zone. It holds them back from speaking openly to friends and family about their challenges. That, to me, is the real shame. Staying too long in the comfort zone leads to a life of inauthenticity, disconnect, and imbalance. To live with vibrant energy, health, and abundance, you need to go where the magic happens. Please do not accept a contracted, smaller version of yourself! You deserve to expand physically, emotionally, and spiritually to be the best you can be.

As a practitioner of both Western and Eastern medicine, I have realized one of the most critical aspects of care involves helping others to open up and reveal whatever their subtle body is holding. When tears appear while speaking to others, I know I'm moving in the right direction.

A doctor's bedside manner illustrates their connection to the patient. Some providers have that connection while others do not. Just as we are guided to connect more deeply with ourselves through the subtle body, we must learn to connect with others on a deeper, more energetic level. To accomplish this, we must allow ourselves to become vulnerable.

Vulnerability is challenging. It risks exposing ourselves in ways that do not feel safe. Yet, in order to become vulnerable, we must trust that the other person is safe to open up to. Trust is risky. If being too trusting in the past left you feeling exposed, criticized, or taken advantage of, it can feel dangerous. I have been there and can empathize with you. Try not to assume that others aren't trustworthy based on previous experiences. Carrying that baggage into your provider's office can create an obstacle to improved health.

To make becoming vulnerable a little easier, look for a friend, provider, family member, significant other, or even a massage therapist who is compassionate and has your best interests in mind. Being vulnerable involves letting others in on your struggles and sharing your feelings about life. It is a mutual sharing, yet done in a very specific way if you are a provider so as not to violate the boundaries of the relationship. Suppose the provider overshares or becomes overly emotional. In that case, this can lead to its own set of challenges, similar in a way to not being vulnerable enough and putting up a wall. It's a delicate balance that ultimately requires compassion from all involved parties—but sometimes sympathy or empathy, precursors to compassion, play a role instead.

THE YOGA JOURNEY

I am grateful that my struggles in medical school led me to begin practicing yoga in my early twenties. As I engaged with yoga and a few other Ayurvedic techniques, I slowly began to notice that I became more compassionate toward myself and others.

What is the purpose of yoga, and how does it foster compassion and empathy?

Yoga has been practiced for centuries by Christians, Hindus, Buddhists, Muslims, atheists, and others. Various religions and cultures have influenced yoga, yet it is not limited to one specific belief system. Yoga comes from the Sanskrit word *yuj,* which means to unify. The practice of yoga allows a connection between mind, body, and spirit. Although most people believe the asanas, or poses, are the central aspect of yoga practice, the truth is, yoga is more about your mind and breath and less about the physical postures.

The *Yoga Sutras of Patanjali,* written by the ancient sage Patanjali about two thousand years ago, consists of 196 verses. This work is considered the foundational guide to the essence of yogic philosophy and practice. Of those 196 verses, *only three verses* discuss the asanas and the postures. The rest focus on how to achieve wisdom and self-realization through yoga.

For this reason, yoga concerns far more than being able to touch your toes. Anyone can practice yoga if it is practiced as it was originally taught, with a focus on mind development. If everyone practiced yoga that way, we would have a much healthier and happier world.

Practicing Yoga the Right Way

There is a right way and a wrong way to practice yoga. If you are currently practicing yoga, evaluate whether your approach benefits your nature, leading to an improvement in your stress personality. Without being mindful of your nature, a yoga practice can do more harm than good. When practiced in alignment with your nature, yoga connects your mind, body, and spiritual self through the regulation of your breath. This enables you to quiet your thoughts and balance your energy body.

The energy body, also referred to as the subtle body, can be likened to a software program. Similar to the way a software program runs the hardware in your computer, the subtle body runs your physical body. Just as software programs have networks of communication to keep the system functioning harmoniously, a network in the subtle body, known as the nadis, keeps your body functioning harmoniously. This system of seventy-two thousand channels carries your life force energy, or prana, throughout your body. If the energy flow is disrupted, you will not feel in harmony. Nadis are similar to the meridians discussed in traditional Chinese medicine. Where Chinese medicine practitioners use acupuncture needles to open up the flow of energy or chi, yoga practitioners use breathwork and postures to improve energy flow.

Yoga has several styles of practices, such as vinyasa (flowing), ashtanga (intense), hatha (balanced), and kundalini (transformational), to name a few. If you were to choose one style of yoga to practice, consider hatha yoga. In Sanskrit, *Ha* refers to the sun, and *Tha* refers to the moon. The polarities of the sun and moon reflect the contradictions within self and in nature. Ha embodies the giving force, which is solar and masculine. It is represented by the rising upon exhalation. Tha reflects the receiving aspect, which is lunar and feminine, represented by the cooling felt upon your inhalation.

Pranayama, or breath control, is an important piece of hatha yoga. *Prana* means life force, and *yama* represents control. The pace of movement is linked to the pace of inhalation and exhalation. Flowing through poses that align with the breath rate creates a natural sense of balance and flow in the body. Practicing controlled breath allows the development of a calmer and more controlled mind, one that is more perceptive and in tune with who you are. This is the epitome of yoga practice: conquering stress and living in greater harmony with yourself. This sense of flow prevents overextension or injury.

Yoga has now been studied extensively, with many studies revealing its beneficial effects on stress, anxiety, and depression.[4] Hatha yoga in particular improves the stress response system in as little as one class![5] For this reason I encourage everyone to experience a hatha yoga class and observe how they feel afterwards. It can shift you quickly.

Four Yogic Paths

As I mentioned earlier, practicing yoga involves more than performing asanas. To unify body, mind, and spirit, you may embark upon yogic paths that have nothing to do with the poses. Ancient texts refer to four yogic paths.

1. Karma yoga is the yogic path of service. Practitioners of karma yoga spend time selflessly serving others. They focus on action to serve their highest purpose and the divine, without concern for recognition or personal gain.

2. Bhakti yoga is the yogic path of devotion. Those who practice bhakti yoga open their hearts to others and the divine. They spend time honoring the divine through bhajans (prayer),

chanting, or performing rituals with an intention to love, surrender, and offer compassion for all living things.

3. Raja yoga is the yogic path of meditation. Practitioners of this path focus on calming the mind through meditation, and they apply the concepts of the eight limbs of yoga taught in *The Yoga Sutras of Patanjali*. This path is most commonly taught in classical yoga classes.

4. Practitioners of jnana yoga, the yogic path of higher wisdom, spend time developing the mind by studying the scriptures, surrounded by enlightened guides who share the teachings. They then apply the teachings to develop a more profound understanding of true nature.

No matter which path or avenue you choose to practice yoga, the final destination is a connection with the self in hopes of reaching a more advanced state of consciousness and awareness.

Whichever journey you choose, if you practice the breath, meditation, asanas, or decide to incorporate one or more of the yogic paths, the natural outcome is cleansing and balancing your subtle body, which encompasses your mind and emotions.

THE CHAKRA SYSTEM

The chakra system is intricately connected to yoga. It lies within the subtle body. Chakra, in Sanskrit, means wheel. The chakra systems consist of spinning energy wheels—vital life force energy centers—that sense and release prana. They are located within the pranamaya kosha or breath layer of the subtle body and carry energy from previous generations (or past lives, based on your beliefs). Ultimately, during yoga practice, this is the energy system being restored.

While the body is said to hold 114 chakras, the seven main chakras running from the base of the spine to the crown of the head are the ones most commonly addressed. Each of these seven chakras links to a neuroendocrine organ in the physical body or annamaya kosha. Chakras communicate through the nadis via a frequency of vibration. Higher chakras spin faster and at a higher frequency than lower ones. Scientific studies have proven measurable electromagnetic emissions from the chakras.[6]

If a chakra becomes blocked, the spin is imbalanced, impacting its vibration. Energy gets stuck, and a feeling of stagnation follows, setting the body up for physical issues. If you become aware of a chakra imbalance, you can take the steps needed to cleanse, energize, and restore balance.

Overall, it is believed that the lower chakras are linked to the physical world and the upper chakras to the spiritual realm. The middle or fourth chakra, the heart chakra, is considered the bridge between them. The lower three chakras—the root, sacral, and solar chakras—relate to your survival nature and your connection to the physical body and material world. These, in my perspective, feed into your reptilian and limbic brain areas. Spending too much of your time connected to those brain areas due to over- or under-expression of the lower chakras, you will find yourself going into a stress state more often and staying there for longer periods.

The higher chakras—the throat, the third eye, and the crown—are linked to a connection to your spiritual self and the divine. These chakras are linked to higher brain functions related to the prefrontal cortex. The heart bridges the lower to the upper chakras. Opening your heart, such as practicing compassion and empathy, allows you to move from reptilian, limbic energy to a more harmonious, prefrontal cortex, blissful energy.

An imbalance in the lower chakras creates the state (windy, fiery, earthy) we discussed in earlier chapters. That ama or toxicity leads to emotional imbalances. Using the Three Brain Optimization Program introduced in chapter 11 to address imbalances in your thinking brain (the mind), feeling brain (ENS), and doing brain (the gut microbiome) moves you from lower chakra vibrational energy to the higher frequency of upper chakra energy.

Focusing on the heart, or bridge chakra, also assists that shift.

The following chart illustrates the progression from the lower to higher chakras, including location and emotional, spiritual, and physical impacts.

Lower Chakras				
Connected with Survival Instincts and the Physical World				
Chakra	Location	Organ	Emotional/ Spiritual Influence	Areas of Physical Impact
Muladhara	Base of spine	Adrenals	Safety, fear, worthiness	Adrenal and lower digestive organs
Svadhisthana	Below navel	Reproductive organs	Sensuality, creativity, trust	Hormonal, urinary, sexual
Manipura	Solar plexus	Above navel, pancreas	Will, confidence, ego, shame, anger	Blood sugar, upper digestive

Heart (Bridge) Chakra				
Transition Between Lower and Higher Chakra Energies				
Chakra	Location	Organ	Emotional/ Spiritual Influence	Areas of Physical Impact
Anahata	Center of chest	Heart	Forgiveness, compassion, self-acceptance	Thymus, immune system, hypertension

Upper Chakras *Connection to Spiritual and Divine Self*				
Chakra	**Location**	**Organ**	**Emotional/ Spiritual Influence**	**Areas of Physical Impact**
Vishuddha	Throat, thyroid	Thymus gland	Speaking your truth and under- standing others	Throat, thyroid
Ajna	Between eyebrows	Pituitary gland	Intuition, higher wisdom	Hormone balance
Sahasrara	Crown of head	Pineal gland, hypothalamus	Connected with all things and the divine	Sleep, migraine, tension headaches

Now, let's take a closer look at each chakra.

The First Chakra: Safety and Security

Located at the base of the spine, the first chakra is known as the muladhara or root chakra. This chakra is linked to feeling stable and grounded, with basic needs met, along with feeling as though you are part of a tribe.

An imbalance here leads to a lack of worthiness, financial troubles, weight issues, or insecurity. This leads to *citta vrtti,* or fluctuations of the mind. An imbalance in the first chakra appears as fear.

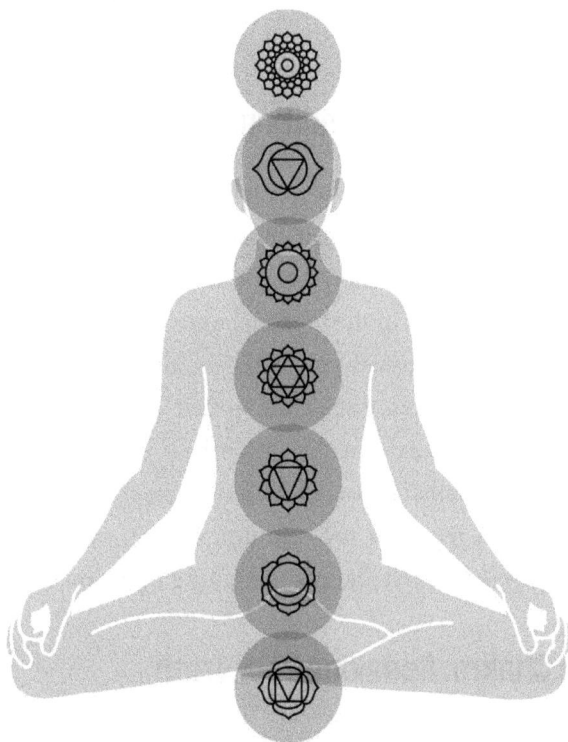

The Second Chakra: Creativity and Sexuality

The second chakra, the svadhisthana or sacral chakra, is located below the belly button. It is linked to emotional stability, pleasure, sensuality, and creativity. An imbalance in the svadhisthana chakra leads to a lack of trust or hurt feelings. Emotional imbalance can occur, expressed by being overly emotional or not emotional enough. A lack of creativity and sexuality imbalances are also common. The emotion here is desire.

The Third Chakra: Personal Power and Self-Esteem

The third chakra, located above the navel, is known as the manipura or solar plexus chakra. It is linked to confidence, willpower, and drive, and therefore, the ego. Self-esteem issues, shame, and feeling either powerless or a sense of arrogance appear with an imbalance in this chakra, and anger is common.

The Fourth Chakra: Unconditional Love

The fourth chakra, located in the center of the chest, is known as the anahata or heart chakra. The heart chakra is linked to unconditional love (true love) toward self and others. It embraces compassion and surrender. An imbalance in the fourth chakra leads to a lack of self-acceptance, feeling hurt, trust issues, loneliness, and an inability to forgive.

Overexpression—and imbalance—often appears in the fourth chakra by sharing love extensively with others yet not taking the time to receive it personally. This chakra is also associated with the thymus gland, which regulates the immune system, specifically T cells. Imbalances here lead to challenges in fighting infections.

The Fifth Chakra: Speaking Your Truth

The fifth chakra, located in the throat region, is known as the vishuddha or throat chakra. It is linked to listening and being heard, communicating, finding one's true voice, and the ability for full and authentic self-expression. When this chakra is balanced, intuition is heard and enables the ability to let others know what one feels, wants, and needs. When it is imbalanced, it may be challenging to speak up, have difficult conversations, or even ask for help. Alternatively, an imbalance may overexpress this chakra, leading to talking too much, too loudly, or too quickly, thus not listening to others.

The fifth chakra is linked to the thyroid gland. Imbalances lead to hypo- or hyperthyroidism, sore throats, and difficulty swallowing.

The Sixth Chakra: Inner Knowing

Located between the eyebrows, this chakra is known as the ajna or third-eye chakra. It is linked to higher intelligence, insight, and being able to discern with mental clarity. This knowing is beyond any gut feelings; it seems as though input is being received from a universal source of wisdom.

This wisdom is always available to us; whether we tap into it is a different story. When the sixth chakra is imbalanced, it may be difficult to connect to intuition due to a reliance on logic or evidence. Clarity is lacking, discernment challenging.

Overexpression in this chakra can result in the development of false beliefs regarding events or situations along with a misguided sense of reality.

The sixth chakra is linked to the pituitary gland, the master hormone regulator. Imbalances in this chakra may lead to imbalanced hormonal regulation. Overexpression can lead to intense dreams, headaches, brow tension, and nightmares.

The Seventh Chakra: Unity and Connection

Also known as the sahasrara or crown chakra, the seventh chakra is located at the crown of the head. This chakra is linked to unity and connection to all things, the belief in synchronicities and divine intervention. You feel blissful, detached, and connected to the divine. When a challenging situation occurs, you believe there is a deeper message or meaning behind it. (Remember the idea of kensho introduced in chapter 8?) There is a sense of non-duality. Imbalance here leads to a feeling that you are not connected to any guidance from a higher power and may become angry, believing that you are not being guided or have to accomplish everything yourself. This chakra is linked to the pineal gland and hypothalamus. Imbalances here lead to sleep issues, challenges with connecting to the circadian rhythm, migraines, and tension headaches.

Working with Chakras

In *Yoga of the Subtle Body*, author and yoga teacher Tias Little writes, "The adrenals are the brain of the lower three chakras, whose intelligence is calibrated to reproduce, defend, and ensure survival."[7]

Most of us experience some imbalance in the first three chakras due to the parental and generational programming that shaped our way of being in the world. Because these chakras are linked to the neuroendocrine organs, the ones that Little referenced, the imbalanced energy flow can lead to hormonal and physical consequences. If the root chakra is imbalanced, it is reflected in a sense of not belonging, lack of self-worth, or not feeling safe, which can lead to excessive adrenal activation. Adrenal imbalances, along with elimination imbalances, are often found when this chakra is not in harmony.

Keep in mind that if one chakra is not resonating at the correct frequency (such as the root), it can imbalance the other chakras. Each chakra can influence the others positively or negatively.

For the second chakra, the sacral chakra, experiencing emotional instability, challenges with enjoying pleasurable activities, and sexual imbalances are linked to challenges in reproductive organs. For women, the resulting hormonal imbalances may manifest as fibroids, abnormal cycles, or endometriosis. In men, it may manifest as poor libido, sexual dysfunction, or even sexual addiction.

A sacral chakra imbalance may be expressed as a lack of power and withholding your will or the egoic imbalances discussed in chapter 11. This may lead to imbalances in the pancreas, which regulates insulin and blood sugar, along with upper digestive issues such as reflux or nausea.

Many people seek tools to tap into a higher spiritual realm and experience a higher vibrational, self-enlightened state. Begin by connecting with the heart chakra, considered the seat of the soul. It serves as a bridge from that material to the spiritual realm.

To enliven the heart chakra, seek love. Right speech—the Buddhist term for nonviolent communication—uses language skills to increase compassion. Listening compassionately, without judgment or criticism, can have a profound effect on yourself and others. Compassion meditation has been shown to lead to changes in brain wave patterns, thus proving you can train yourself to be compassionate.[8]

Bhujangasana, otherwise known as the cobra pose, is one of the most beneficial for opening and balancing the heart chakra. A variety of methods can be utilized to balance the chakras, especially the lower three, such as specific pranayama (breath) exercises, yoga poses, essential oils, and even mantras. A regular, daily routine is fundamental to reducing stress and balancing adrenal function while stabilizing the chakras.

A routine connects with the circadian pattern and sets the energy body on the right course for the day. When the sun rises, light enters the brain through the eyes. It activates the pineal gland, telling it to turn off melatonin production, thus allowing cortisol levels to rise. That wakes you up and gets you ready for the day. Through that process, the anja chakra—your intuitive third eye—becomes activated. Waking up at the same time daily activates the hypothalamic-pituitary axis to harmonize endocrine function and regulate your system. (And remember: the hypothalamus is your divine internal mother!)

TAKE-HOME POINTS

1. Your symptoms are a message that your body, both physical and subtle, is not in balance. Listen to those messages and take action to shift your state and your lifestyle.

2. Excess vata (windy) energy can lead to a freeze state, leading to neck pain, headaches, an anxious mind, and constipation.

3. Suppression or repression of emotions is common, and it effects the physical body when stored in the subtle body for too long.

4. Vulnerability is one step toward developing meaningful relationships. Trust can be established once you are vulnerable to allowing another person in.

5. Compassion means "to suffer together." Empathy improves connection and allows compassion to emerge. Sympathy, a pity-based response, furthers disconnection.

6. Yoga comes from a Sanskrit word meaning *to yoke* or *to unite*. The practice of yoga is meant to unify you with your higher self.

7. The practice of yoga is more about the regulation of your mind than it is about doing the poses.

8. Hatha yoga incorporates the concept of embodying movements with the breath, thus aligning your asanas (or poses) with yourself.

9. There are four yogic paths: karma (service), bhakti (devotion), raja (meditation), and jnana (higher wisdom).

10. The chakras are located in the subtle body and carry the emotional blueprint of your past. Chakra health is dictated by the emotional and thought-pattern energy you carry.

11. Cleansing and harmonizing the chakras to an optimal state allows you to feel better energetically, emotionally, and physically.

12. The lower three chakras are often imbalanced. The heart chakra may bridge the lower chakras and move you into the higher chakras linked to the spiritual, higher mind realm.

ACTION STEPS

Throughout your life, have you had anyone tune in and check in with you about various impactful events and allow you to process them? Take some time now to journal about any experiences where another person either allowed you to become vulnerable or prevented you from it.

If you have been able to connect to your emotions and tie them to your physiology, allow yourself to journal about these questions, ideally in a relaxed state first thing in the morning when you can free-flow your thoughts.

- Where does emotion appear in your body?

- What is the emotion?

- Think of the primary emotions of fear, sadness, anger, shame, pride, and disgust. What is the message behind each emotion?

13

Stepping Out of the Comfort Zone

"Our deepest fear is not that we are inadequate, our deepest fear is that
we are powerful beyond measure. It is our light, not our darkness,
that most frightens us."
—Marianne Williamson

I'll never forget the conversation I had with the outgoing chief resident of neurology. We were out to lunch at a nice Thai restaurant close to the training hospital where we both worked. As I enjoyed my pad thai noodles, she described my responsibilities as the new chief resident. I would be in charge of the call schedule, carry a twenty-four-seven pager when I covered Christ Hospital, and would be responsible for meeting with department and program chairs regularly to ensure the program was running smoothly.

She then asked me what I planned on researching for my senior paper, one of the requirements of my training. After deciding on specializing in headache medicine, I told her I wanted to write a review paper on Botulinum toxin type A, otherwise known as Botox®, and its outcomes with headaches and migraines.

A look of surprise and disgust crossed her face. "Why would you write a paper on that?" she exclaimed. "Do you know if it turns out to be a placebo, you will be mocked? It will be hard to recover from that! Especially because this is your first paper."

I paused, a slightly queasy but familiar sensation rolling through my stomach. It was my body telling me I didn't align with the situation in front of me. It was the same feeling I'd had when I was offered Prozac® for my "depression." This time, however, I was older and wiser. Although I knew she was trying to protect me from what others would say, I frankly didn't care. I stopped caring what others thought years before, and I now had years of medical training and residency programs under my belt. I trusted my intuition, as it had a good record of guiding me in the right direction.

I thanked her for her feedback and told her I was planning on writing the paper anyway, even if it turned out to be a sham procedure. In the end, the paper was written and published. After eight years of injecting the toxin without FDA approval—off-label, as we call it in the medical world—this drug finally reached approval due to its highly beneficial responses for those with chronic migraines. Patients were able to taper off their daily prescription medications, reducing their as-needed meds. They finally experienced migraines that were less frequent, less severe, and more treatable.

During a time when Vicodin®, a medication with potential for addiction, was being prescribed for migraines, I was grateful for an alternative. Tuning into my gut allowed me to deliver Botox® for years before its effectiveness was recognized by the mainstream. I was also able to share its impact with others before it was approved, thus advancing awareness of this novel approach and its expanded use. Eventually, I became a speaker and trainer for those administering Botox® injections for migraine and one of the nation's experts on the procedure.

Why did this happen?

The answer lies in being comfortable with the uncomfortable. It lies in trusting your inner knowing more than your intellect, which is guided by data, evidence, and science. I found myself stepping out of my comfort zone, trusting the process, and taking a chance to study something novel. I was uncertain. I risked mockery and damage to my reputation if it did not work. Thankfully, an outstanding physician whom I worked for encouraged me to take the step. That physician helped me finalize and publish the paper. That support and my intuition were all I needed. I am glad I let my intuition be my guide, not only to do the research but also to offer it to patients struggling with pain.

When it comes to speaking your truth or taking actions that may make you uneasy, why do so many hold back? What prevents you from moving into the place where magic happens?

After many years of enduring my own discomfort with living my truth, and working with coaching clients also challenged by it, I recognized a similar theme. It begins with a sense of excitement or inspiration about a novel idea and a rush of endorphins from imagining the possibility. Then, the emotional brain moves to the lower chakra energy of fear and shame. Potential risks are perceived, and other unpleasant emotions arise. This engages the prefrontal cortex and triggers a thinking pattern that emphasizes staying safe, avoiding risk, and remaining in the comfort zone.

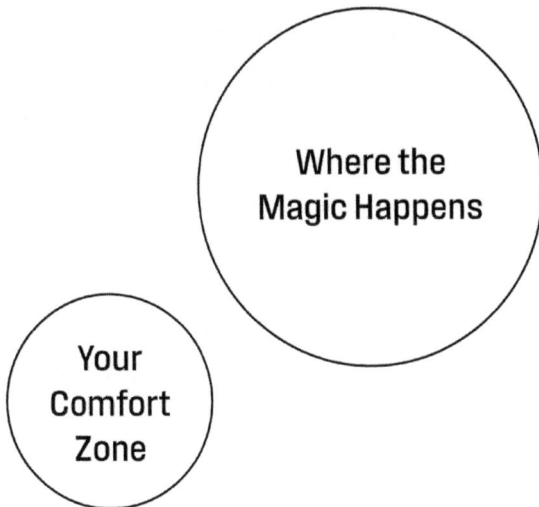

Where the
Magic Happens

Your
Comfort
Zone

As the excitement fades, questions arise. What if I fail? What if I am mocked? What if it doesn't work out?

The "what-iffing" begins and just doesn't stop. Your first brain holds this pattern of questioning and immobilizes you.

OBSTACLES AND YOUR DHARMA

Obstacles to growth can be internal or external. Internal obstacles are the inner programs, thoughts, beliefs, and views that block you from being your truest, most authentic self. External obstacles are situations outside yourself that prevent you from living authentically, such as a significant other or parent who tells you that you will never be able to accomplish the task.

Here is the truth: everyone I have met on this journey has obstacles. That is why they are stuck! Discover your obstacles and clear them so that you can live in your highest state. In Eastern medicine, living at your full potential is living your dharma, your unique offering to this world, and it is your duty to share this with others.

My mother was the most incredible cook. She created delectable meals, and she was revered by many of our family and friends for her skills. Cooking was my mom's dharma. When she began to struggle with her brain health and stopped cooking, we all felt the loss.

Your ability to fulfill your dharma affects everyone around you. You serve others by living your dharma. At some level, the pursuit of dharma is a selfless act where you can make this world a better place simply by being the highest version of yourself. It serves you as well; when living in your dharma, you will feel blissful and healthy.

How beautiful would it be if everyone lived according to this principle?

I delved way out of my comfort zone into the area of gut-brain science when my dear daughter, Ariya, began having headaches at the age of five. After deciding to test her for food intolerances, I attended a weekend functional medicine conference for training on allergy testing and interpreting the results. We found that she was severely gluten, dairy, and egg intolerant. Due to my heavy clinic schedule and the easy availability of the traditional Western diet, those seemed to be the only foods I fed her at that age. I often purchased items with many of these ingredients. This was in 2007, when almond and other non-dairy milks were not a thing. Her physician said that she would suffer from bone loss if I stopped giving her cow's milk. I would be going against medical advice if we chose to go down that path.

We went anyway.

We now have data showing that cow-based milk may not reduce fractures as once believed. For some people, cow's milk is inflammatory, thus increasing their risk for fracture.[1]

Even though prevailing medical opinion was an external obstacle to implementing a dietary change for my daughter, I stepped out of my comfort zone and lived into my dharma: helping people heal. I placed Ariya on a modified diet to eliminate triggering foods, and magic happened. Feel free to read more about her journey in my first book, *The Mysterious Mind*.*

Now, fifteen years later, Ariya remains headache-free due to the interventions we chose when she was five. After strengthening her digestive system, she returned to the foods that had once troubled her. She has a healthy body and a strong mind. She recently noticed that avoiding gluten had a positive impact on her immune system, which was impacted during pandemic challenges. She follows her intuition regarding her diet based on her current physiology, environmental stressors, and lifestyle. I am grateful she has the knowledge and tools to improve her physiology and empower herself. This is the magic I am referring to.

Certain moments in your life define you. Moments that, at the time, may seem inconsequential. My bout with insomnia was one of

---

* Ariya's story appears in chapter 5 of *The Mysterious Mind*, "The Gut Brain Link," page 53.

those moments, as was Ariya's journey with headaches. It would take me years to understand this idea of transformational moments and the Japanese Zen concept of kensho.

Kensho, as you may recall, means "seeing one's true nature." I expand it to include seeing the true nature of our experience. Once we understand the nature of self, we can expand to understand the nature of experience. I have had many kensho moments. When these moments happen, they stop me and give me no choice but to pause and reflect.

When you encounter a kensho moment, instead of asking why this is happening *to* you, ask why this is happening *for* you. That shift draws you into growth rather than becoming a victim of life and circumstances. Pause, reflect on the situation at hand, and grow from it by shifting some aspect of yourself or your life.

When I was stuck, I had been living with such drive and intensity that I never took the time to pause and reflect on my *why*. I never even gave myself a chance to know myself. I was too busy moving to think. I spent time outward and rarely went in. I had no idea who I was or where I was going. I simply knew that I felt uncomfortable if I was not continually productive. Staying "on" and active allowed me to feel purposeful. Yet, in the end, I realized that rushing forward with no insight or direction leads nowhere but stuck, unhappy, and unsatisfied.

CHOOSE YOUR DESTINATION

Close your eyes for a moment and imagine where you would like to be in three years. Engage your senses and ask yourself what you see, feel, and hear in that environment. How will you know when you have arrived at your *final destination*?

If you are currently experiencing tremendous stress, digestive symptoms, headaches, and autoimmune or mental health issues, it may feel overwhelming to think that far ahead. In that case, instead of imagining your final destination, picture where you would like to be along the path toward it in one month or three. Or imagine how you will feel and live when one facet of your health improves, then another. Picture your anticipated results as deeply and vividly as possible without creating a sense of overwhelm. This is your vision; this is your journey.

Notice I am encouraging you to imagine yourself moving *toward an outcome* instead of *away from the present*. Instead of saying, "I have to get rid of my migraines," or "I would like to reduce *x*, *y*, or *z* in my life," try, "I believe I can experience pain freedom," or whatever else you would like to bring into your life. We often hear people say they need to see something to believe it. I invite you to first believe it, and then, I promise, you will see it.

Creating a receptive state allows your brain to focus on a pain-free or higher aspiration state, allowing you to move in that direction and manifest your goals. The universe doesn't give you what you *want*; instead, the universe reflects *who you are*. If you do not like what you see, the onus is on you to shift your belief system.

It sounds simple, and it isn't always easy to make that shift, yet I have seen it powerfully transform many people.

After establishing a firm belief that your desired outcome is possible and moving toward that belief, establish clarity about what you want. Think of it like ordering food from a menu. When you arrive at the restaurant and clearly list your choices to the waiter, you receive a dish that matches what you ordered. If you are unsure and focus on items you do not want, you'll never receive what you do want. That is the idea of goal-setting. Visualize what you want and move toward your final destination.

After reading *The 7 Habits of Highly Effective People* back in my twenties, I felt empowered by concepts that would allow me to be more successful in life.[2] As I incorporated these seven habits into my way of living, I understood my thoughts could influence my outcomes in life.

The second habit was the most profound for me: "Begin with the end in mind." This is not a sad or morbid perspective that focuses on death instead of life. It's quite the opposite. If anything, being mindful of any journey's conclusion enables you to be more aware of the present moment.

When prescribing short-acting meds to reduce pain for patients experiencing migraine, I encourage them to remain mindful of their condition and the potential consequences of long-term, frequent usage. To help them understand, I ask how they would feel in a month's time if they started a practice of getting to bed on time nightly. Anticipation is the first step toward knowing what your end goals are so you can live each day with more presence and connection to the moment.

As I pursued my training in neurolinguistic programming, otherwise known as NLP, I was fascinated with the practice's origins. The founders, Richard Bandler and John Grinder, studied the thoughts and language patterns of successful people. Then, they developed a model to understand their techniques and apply them to daily life. It became clear that success could be achieved by individuals who considered how they thought, perceived the world, and used language to describe life's experiences.

For more than two decades, I observed thousands of individuals and noted which patients succeeded and which ones did not. Those who succeeded had inner programs that worked for them. Those who did not succeed had programs that work against them. Anyone moving toward a goal needs to clear any baggage holding them back. Once that baggage is cleared—for some, that means trauma—they can freely move toward their goal. Obtaining mental and spiritual health leads to physical health. In this way, whole brain and body intelligence leads to a balance of mind, body, and spirit.

To do this, you want to start by thinking about your attention, intention, and meaning (AIM) and your avatar.

Your AIM is your North Star, the direction you plan to go. It is based on where you are now and who you would like to be in the future. Your AIM can continue to change over time as your life path changes and you evolve. Who do you want to serve? Who is your tribe when it comes to your career, your friends, and even your family?

Choosing the area of life that challenges you the most is the best place to start.

Your avatar is your jivatman, your soul, or your higher/ideal self. You will never shift from this self. It is the true you. How does your avatar look, feel, and think? What does your avatar genuinely want to accomplish in life?

ASSESSING PHYSICAL HEALTH

Now, let's move from mind and spiritual health to physical health. Many clients ask how best to assess themselves in terms of their current physical state when there are minimal symptoms or no disease to diagnosis. This is one of the most important questions to ask. Don't wait until disease sets in to start taking your health seriously. One of the best ways to assess your current state is by obtaining straightforward labs. These can be done with your primary care physician. Consider reviewing *The Mysterious Mind*, Chapter 4, "Understanding Your Body's Biochemistry."[3] In that chapter, we delve into the intricate process of understanding your physiology from a clinical perspective, unraveling the complexities of your body's functioning.

Do not believe you are fine just because your labs are normal. Remember what I was told back in the day as I struggled with severe insomnia? I was certainly not feeling fine despite "normal" labs. I am glad I embarked upon functional medicine and Ayurvedic training to learn what truly optimal function means in terms of labs and physiology: having labs in the mid-range of normal along with a sense of energetic balance.

For example, if your doctor finds you have a vitamin D level of 34 (a healthy range is considered 30 to 100), he or she may report that your labs are normal. But what if you are experiencing neck tightness and fatigue? Vitamin D plays a key role in inflammatory pathways. In fact, it behaves more like a hormone than a vitamin. It regulates the expression of hundreds of genes involved in skeletal and biological functions. Thus, if you have neck pain and headaches or cardiovascular or immune system struggles, a higher vitamin D level may be beneficial to you. I wish it were easy to improve D3 levels by spending more time in the sun, but unfortunately, it's far more complicated than a trip to the beach. Understanding your low vitamin D requires looking into WHY it is low in the first place.

Recent studies reveal that vitamin D plays a role in maintaining a healthy microbiome too. Dysbiosis, an unhealthy bacterial balance in the gut, is now believed to be linked to low levels of vitamin D.[4] Are you struggling with dysbiosis? Vitamin D can help repair your gut lining, and studies have shown that vitamin D improves the diversity of bacteria in your gut.[5]

Anxiety and depression may also be linked to low vitamin D levels.[6]

The pivotal labs I encourage most to obtain, at a minimum, are the comprehensive metabolic panel, the complete blood count, vitamin D levels, fasting cholesterol, free thyroid levels, ferritin level, and HbA1c (blood sugar).**

Interpreting labs can be a challenging task, yet once you begin to understand the meaning behind the numbers and see the labs as a marker of your mind, body, and spiritual health, you can use them to help you improve your lifestyle and even prevent the disease from occurring in the first place.

I have recommended supplements for over two decades. I have even compounded my own nutrient and Ayurvedic blends, along with offering tailored IV nutrient therapy in my practice. But please be mindful; adding supplements should be done under the supervision

---

** If you are seeking deeper understanding of your labs, review *The Mysterious Mind*, chapter 4, "Understanding your Body's Body Chemistry" for information on cholesterol, hormones and other labs and chapter 6, "Adrenal Fatigue: A Hidden Pervasive Syndrome" to learn more about adrenal-thyroid pathways.

of someone who has experience utilizing various supplements in their clinical practice for years. It is crucial to monitor the outcomes of different protocols, recheck labs, and match the results to your symptoms periodically. The goal is to use supplements to balance the doshas, the stress personality, and create a harmonious system.

I recommend investing more energy in digestive health. Tests for gut issues have become more specific and reliable over the years. Food intolerance testing and microbiome testing, based on individual needs, indicate foods that harm the gut. Simply removing the food alone will not provide healing. Eliminating harmful foods should be done while balancing the three brains. You must shift the thinking and emotions that went along with the development of the intolerance. In that way, you may be able to reintroduce the food later in your journey. Intolerances can change over time.

Remember, how you process your thoughts and emotions (in your first and second brain, respectively) affects how you process foods. If your mind program keeps you in an anxious or angry thinking and feeling state, it will affect microbiome health.

Most people become upset about what they need to remove from the diet. I encourage an abundance versus scarcity mindset. Imagining replacement foods creates a completely different outlook that can open you to new foods, spices, and even teas to balance gut health.

These approaches, along with adding essential medical-grade supplements, will repair a gut that may be leaky.

LEAKY GUT AND LEAKY BRAIN

Leaky gut, also referred to as increased intestinal permeability, damages the integrity of your digestive lining. It becomes impaired due to stress, toxins, a poor diet, poorly digested foods, or poor eating habits, and it is believed to be present in 80 to 90 percent of Americans. For years, it was not considered to be a legitimate pathological process. Yet, recent studies clearly define it as a valid entity that can impact many conditions.[7]

Having a leaky gut perpetuates more food intolerances. Inflammatory reactions at the gut level are measured by secretory IgA, a protective antibody in the gut. This antibody binds and neutralizes an endotoxin known as lipopolysaccharide (LPS), which is the breakdown product of the outer wall of certain bacteria. Then, this endotoxin is cleared out of the system during the natural elimination process.

We all have LPS. The challenge arises when it moves from within the gut lumen (essentially, the lining) and enters the systemic circulation. This can happen when certain keystone gut bacteria are lost due to stress, toxins, and certain foods, as mentioned above, and the production of tight junction proteins is reduced. These proteins keep the endothelial cells together, allowing the gut membrane to remain intact.

To make matters worse, with a shift in gut integrity, IgA production may be impaired. The combination of these factors prevents toxic LPS from being neutralized, allowing them to float freely in their toxic form. LPS can then leak into the systemic circulation and create a host of inflammatory reactions throughout the body.

Most people do not realize they have a leaky gut. I didn't know I had one until I did the testing—and I am one of the healthiest eaters I know! I regularly eliminate the first thing in the morning upon awakening. Even when we hiked up to Machu Picchu over four strenuous days, I was able to have a daily elimination. With the help of some Ayurvedic gut-balancing herbals, at the crack of dawn in a stinky outhouse, I would squat and eliminate in a matter of two minutes. Others in my group were not able to accomplish this. The stress of the trek led to a halt in elimination. You may notice this happening when you fly. Some patients report that travel or stress constipates them.

I manage to preserve harmony when I travel. This is partly due to my focus on maintaining gut health between my travels, preparing before travel, and years of taking Ayurvedic, home-cooked meals to work. As much as I am able, I focus on eating three solid meals per day without multitasking and while sitting. In the past, I was told that I was being difficult or demanding when I asked for a lunch break or to sit while I ate. That was not my intention. I simply have boundaries essential to my well-being.

I value a healthy eating routine. While I occasionally order sushi or another somewhat healthy equivalent, most of the time, I eat home-cooked foods prepared with whole foods, properly spiced, and derived from Mother Nature. I am grateful to have help from my mother-in-law, who cooks for our family twice a week. In addition, I rarely ate dinner late at night.

Sitting down at every meal is very important. I have been known to go to parties and ask a friend to sit with me to avoid standing while eating. Why is that important? The simple act of standing tells the brain you are in danger, and blood flow shifts from your stomach to your legs, preparing you to run from that proverbial bear.

How many of you follow all the rules I mentioned above?

If you don't—which I suspect is true for the majority of you—you are at high risk for leaky gut. If that's the case, I recommend some life-style changes.

As mentioned before, gut impacts are often top-down, with first brain and second brain thoughts and emotions affecting the third brain or gut. A leaky gut shows up insidiously and often without any obvious symptoms. The gut slowly shifts over time, starting with a shift in healthy populations of bacteria, especially a reduction of the keystone bacteria that do most of the internal maintenance and housekeeping.

Then, the integrity of the gut lining erodes as subtle signs of inflammation appear, starting at the gut level and moving to the rest of the body. You may notice your neck getting tighter or the development of occasional headaches, skin rashes or acne, occasional constipation or reflux, abnormal menstrual cycles, forgetfulness, feeling distracted or anxious, and the list goes on.

I have met many people who tell me they felt fine until suddenly they weren't. It wasn't sudden, I promise you. Unfortunately, the gut allows a silent attack on your body without you even knowing. This process alone can lead to an activated adrenal system, moving you into a windy, fiery, or earthy state. Even the state change may begin subtly. You and others around you may not notice your slight anxiety, irritability, or lower moods unless paying close attention. The gut moves into a state known as basal inflammation. In this state, the gut produces inflammatory cytokines. These cytokines, or inflammatory proteins, are linked to insomnia, psoriasis, and autoimmune disorders, along with other conditions.[8]

THE LAWS OF NATURE

The story of your journey to health has a beautiful ending. You are living in a time with access to novel and ancient methods for improvement. The body is always in the process of tissue and muscle rebuilding (anabolic state) and breakdown (catabolic state). The goal is to not spend too much time in the catabolic, a.k.a. aging, pathway.

The Steroid Hormone Pathway:
It All Begins With Cholestrol (Figure 4)

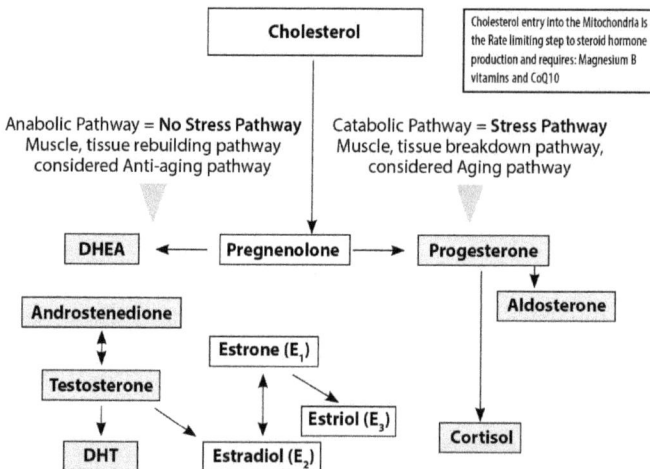

Cholesterol, after converting to pregnenolone, has a choice to enter the anabolic pathway or the catabolic pathway based on the needs of each of our cells and our body's requirements at that moment.

Even though I have encouraged you not to *over* stress, please remember that the appropriate amount of stress is good for you. A certain level of short-lived stress helps the system strengthen. This is known as *hormesis*. The stressor stimulates the body to manufacture more mitochondria, which regulates the energy system. It is only when the exposure or perception of stress extends beyond the system's ability to handle it that the body enters an excessive catabolic state. This can occur if you don't take breaks from work or exercise, if you indulge in too many cold plunges, or even if you fast too frequently.

In the catabolic state, not only will you age faster, you may also enter perimenopause or even stop cycling at an earlier age and develop diseases earlier that are potentially more challenging to treat. With a few simple yet powerful steps, you can shift from your aging, stressed, and catabolic state into an antiaging, restorative, and anabolic one.

Yes, it really can be done. Ayurveda, which is the wisdom of healing, or the science of longevity, focuses on prevention and reduction in disease manifestation by addressing energy imbalances before they lead to physical ones.

A few of the key solutions involve reconnecting with nature's cycles and aligning your body with the sun and the moon. Another principle is to use food to shift you into an antiaging, more harmonized mind and body state. According to Ayurveda, with a poor diet, medicine is of no need. With a good diet, medicine is of no use.

We all have longevity signals that become activated as we follow certain laws of nature. These are scripted in ancient science. Ayurveda encourages eating according to daylight patterns. Agni or digestive fire is lower in the morning when the sun is lower in the sky, so a light breakfast is recommended. However, at noon, when the sun is at its peak, the body makes the highest level of digestive enzymes. Therefore, lunch is believed to be the most important—and the largest—meal of the day. Later, as the sun sets, the production of digestive enzymes and hydrochloric acid declines. It is difficult for the gut to digest a bigger meal later in the evening. Dinner is not usually eaten until after 7:00

p.m. to permit a fasting state between dinner and breakfast. Healthy mealtimes are a matter of aligning with the circadian rhythm and tuning yourself into your natural digestive process.

It is important to have on time and off time for eating too. These days, intermittent fasting is met with enthusiasm as a novel concept. However, it has been discussed in ancient literature for thousands of years. I am glad now it is finally getting the recognition it deserves. Science is now backing this up. Fasting is one of the most beneficial things you can do for your health. When you fast, you increase stem cell production and induce autophagy, a process of cleansing harmful cells. This process leads to a reduction in inflammation and moves you into an antiaging state. It inhibits the mTOR gene controlling the mTOR pathway, which is involved in cellular growth linked to aging and diseases such as cancer.[9] Fasting plays an incredible role in suppressing this gene.

For an optimal digestive system, your gut must align with the cycles of day and night. This function is mainly directed by the hypothalamus, the circadian pacemaker of the brain (or divine mother). The hypothalamus should signal you to eat based on hunger signals. You eat, then allow your gut to process the food and cleanse it to prepare for the next meal.

When you are not eating, your migratory motor complex (MMC) goes into action to strengthen and reset the gut. If you eat continuously, you may weaken your digestive strength and MMC. Fasting with the season change, which has been recommended in Ayurveda for thousands of years, is now proven to be medically beneficial. These "secrets" encourage longevity and graceful aging.

SUPPLEMENTS, MEDICATIONS, AND YOUR GUT

As mentioned earlier, please only add supplements under provider supervision. Digestive supplements are often the most beneficial to start with. They tend to offer the fastest relief of symptoms when used wisely and with appropriate monitoring. Based on clinical studies and my personal experience working with thousands of patients over the years, I have found that certain types of probiotics and digestive herbals are more effective than others.

We now are learning about new classes of supplements known as psychobiotics, which improve brain health and mental well-being by improving microbial balance. Some of these psychobiotics even modulate the stress response system, reducing cortisol, perceived stress, and pro-inflammatory cytokines.[10]

Medications impact your system more than you may realize. One round of antibiotics leads to dysbiosis (abnormal growth of bacteria) and shifts the diversity of bacteria, which may take months to recover from.[11] It is now clear that over-the-counter medications such as ibuprofen and naproxen (brand names Advil and Aleve) wreak havoc on your digestive lining, increasing your risk of ulcers, gastritis, and bleeding. Excessive use of acetaminophen (brand name Tylenol) has become the number one cause of liver transplants. Due to this, a label change reduced the maximum acetaminophen dosage per tablet to 325 mg to reduce the risk to the liver.[12]

Other common medications known to affect digestive function include steroids, certain blood pressure medications, and antidepressants. Newer medications for migraine, the calcitonin gene-related peptide (CGRP) antagonists, also influence the digestive system in ways that are still being discovered. Protein pump inhibitors and other acid blockers may lead to secondary issues, such as impaired magnesium absorption, potentially leading to arrhythmias, muscle spasms, or seizures[13] along with impairment of B12 and vitamin D absorption.[14]

According to ancient wisdom, suppressing the system from a natural function, such as blocking the production of stomach acid, may worsen the original symptom or even create newer, unrelated symptoms. This is proven by modern science. Recent data shows that acid blockers over time may lead to an impairment of kidney function.[15]

Your body is trying to send you a message with symptoms. If you are not listening or ignore any symptom by suppressing it, the body's message grows louder until you have no choice but to respond. I have witnessed this time and time again.

DIVERSITY AND YOUR HEALTH

Finding internal alignment by balancing your thoughts, creating coherence with your brain regions, and generating harmony in your physical body require attention to the areas asking for support and utilizing the best available tools to provide that support.

Often what is missing is something that may be unexpected: diversity.

Humans crave diversity, and diversity benefits us in many ways. When I ran the integrative center years ago, having a front desk person who could greet the patients, perform an intake for my patients, and also order products for our apothecary when our inventory was low was key to our survival as a center. We trained all our team members to multitask, so we were never in a pinch if someone didn't show up for work.

I entered business school as an undergraduate student at the University of Illinois in Urbana-Champaign. After a year, I craved science, so I ended up leaving business school. I switched to liberal arts and sciences and focused on two majors, economics and biology. Little did I realize how impactful that would be for me. As I diversified my exposure and stimulated my right-sided, creative brain with economics classes, I juxtaposed this with biology classes, which stimulated my left-sided, logical brain. I made friends who were polar opposites. The business students tended to be more relaxed and sociable, while the biology students were more academic and serious. This allowed me to develop all aspects of my personality. As I spent time with my unique circles of friends, I exposed myself to a more diverse cuisine too. My business school friends enjoyed grilled foods and pasta dishes. My science friends tended to favor ethnic cuisines.

Eventually, by experiencing diversity in career, friends, food, and thoughts, resistance to differences and change is reduced, moving you beyond your comfort zone. Diversity allows brain hemispheres to balance and obtain coherence. Brain coherence moves you into a more balanced, energetic state, which is optimal for your nature. As the brain achieves coherence, so does the body. Whole-brain and whole-body coherence leads to the reduction of disease, stress, overwhelm, anxiety, and poor health, moving you into focus, clarity, and happiness with abundant energy and health.

This is how this looks:

Diversity of Friends → Diversity of Thoughts → Diversity of Experiences → Diversity of Foods → Reduced Resistance = Balanced Brain Right to Left, Front to Back, Top and Down!

Concepts from ancient wisdom will help you achieve a healthy digestive lining with a balanced microbiome and third brain. Eat what Mother Nature has given you and utilize spices with each meal. The six tastes—sweet, sour, salty, bitter, spicy, and astringent—should be incorporated into each meal. Spices, along with a wide range of cuisines, enhance microbial diversity. Spices not only help with microbial diversity but also, because they contain phytochemicals such as flavonoids and polyphenols, they may have protective effects on aging and even prevent Alzheimer's disease.[16] When you lack diversity, you are at higher risk for diseases such as diabetes, eczema, and obesity—just to name a few.

You may think that eating exotic foods and incorporating spices is too challenging. It is not as hard to do as you think. Adding unique ingredients and spices to your current cuisine can make all the difference. Shifting to the best quality and type of proteins, carbohydrates, and oils, and adding a few spices will transform your meals into Ayurvedic ones, thus balancing your stress personality type.

In addition, it is important to offer some type of hormesis to your gut. The Ayurvedic diet encourages the consumption of lectins in your cuisine. Lectins are found in tomatoes, beans, lentils, nightshade vegetables, and rice, to name a few. Unfortunately, a few modern thinkers are perpetuating the belief that lectins should be avoided in everyone's diet. This is entirely untrue. Some people may be sensitive to lectins, and that I can appreciate. Choosing the correct form of lectins, in the ideal amount, while preparing them optimally may be necessary for your system to tolerate and benefit from them.

What are lectins, you may ask? Lectins are proteins that bind to carbohydrates. I have had patients ask me over the years if lectins were bad for them. Let me ask you this: if Mother Nature placed lectins in our foods, do you not think that was done for a reason?

Lectin slows down digestion. It lowers the glycemic index (diabetes-causing) effect of the carbohydrate you are consuming. Suppose you avoid these foods regularly without being clinically monitored. In that case, you won't receive the beneficial effects of these foods, which include reducing your risk of heart disease, cancer, and even neurodegenerative diseases. Avoidance may actually cause harm. Removing these foods from the diet risks the eventual development of a fragile digestive system that becomes more vulnerable to these ingredients. Simply learning how to prepare lectins, along with incorporating spices, allows you to enjoy them and embrace their health-promoting benefits.

TAKE-HOME POINTS

1. Staying in your comfort zone leads to potential feelings of disconnect, overwhelm, and feeling stuck in life.

2. Enthusiasm to move in a new direction may be compromised by unconscious emotional programs such as shame, guilt, fear,

and anger, which prevent you from stepping into the zone where magic happens.

3. Living in alignment with your purpose, or dharma, often requires moving past both internal and external obstacles.

4. Kensho experiences are often seen as challenges, yet they are opportunities to move into growth versus becoming a victim of the circumstances of your life.

5. Moving toward what you want rather than away from what you do not is an empowering shift in perspective. It will help the universe assist you with accomplishing your goals.

6. Knowing your AIM and avatar will guide you toward your ideal end goals, leading to mind and spiritual health.

7. Evaluating labs in conjunction with your energetic self allows individualized guidance for improved health based on your unique symptoms. Labs that are in the "normal" range may not be optimal for you.

8. Along with the evaluation of your physical body, food intolerance testing and microbiome testing can provide insights into healing a leaky gut and creating harmony in your first and second brains.

9. Leaky gut is linked to inflammatory conditions in the body.

10. Psychobiotics are novel probiotics that may reduce stress, cortisol production, and even pro-inflammatory cytokines.

11. If you start a protocol of supplements or dietary or lifestyle changes, do so only under provider supervision so you can align these elements to your specific needs.

12. Medications can lead to imbalances in the microbiome.

13. Diversity of individuals, experiences, and even foods allow you to be healthier, more balanced, and evolve into the best version of yourself.

14. Toxic foods, friends, and experiences keep you stuck in a pattern. Clearing toxicity from your life is the first step toward healing.

ACTION STEPS

Grab a journal and answer the following questions:

- Where do you struggle the most? Is it in your career, health, relationships, or family?

- Do you have toxicity in your life?

- They may speak negatively, gossip, or critique you or others. Do they not respect you or value what you offer in this world?

- Are they jealous or envious of you or others?

- When it comes to foods, do you eat toxic foods or foods that do not align with your stress state? Do you eat foods that are processed and laden with artificial ingredients?

- With your career, ask yourself if you have a job you love or have high pressure, demanding deadlines, are not getting paid enough, or feel unworthy.

- Are you holding onto mental toxins?

- Do you have toxic thoughts about someone you fought with in your early years?

- Do you have toxic feelings about a relationship that ended badly?

Now that you have written down all your toxic situations, spend some time processing what that means for you.

14

The Next Steps on Your Journey

"I have feet in my shoes, now where will I go?"
—*Dr. Seuss*

The true purpose of this book is to share my vulnerable journey, from a sleepless medical student on the verge of quitting to an evolved physician and coach. Along this path, I discovered tools that seemed radical at the time but ultimately empowered me to heal and overcome. As Robert Frost would say, I took the road less traveled, and it made all the difference. This journey transformed my fear into courage, despair into hope, and darkness into light. These insights not only changed my life and the lives of my family but also allowed me to inspire patients, clients, friends, and colleagues to shift how they approach their lives.

Our current health care system is broken, and it's clear that integrating emotional health with physical health is essential. We must recognize the mind-body connection and understand how subtle, energetic influences play a crucial role in healing. By enhancing the prefrontal cortex (PFC) and reducing the input from the reptilian and limbic systems, we can find more peace within ourselves. This shift occurs when we delve into understanding our stress personality, uncover why we're at odds with ourselves, and use ancient tools to resolve this inner conflict.

It's not just about identifying imbalances in vata, pitta, or kapha energies but also taking the time to understand how we arrived there and why we remain in an unbalanced state. As you observe your stress personality, which unconsciously protects you from perceived danger, techniques like reverse nostril breathing can harmonize the right and left hemispheres of the brain, easing the overactive reptilian response. These simple breathwork practices, especially when combined with movement, help clear toxins and open the subtle energy flow within, allowing you to shift from a stuck, restricted state to one that's more content, peaceful, and vibrant.

Understanding the stories you tell yourself can lead to profound changes in how you experience life. If you struggle with health, career, friendships, or family, it's worth reevaluating the beliefs you hold in these areas. As you change your story, your life transforms. You become more aligned with your inner wisdom, and your intellect sharpens, allowing you to make wiser decisions. The mistakes of the intellect become a thing of the past as you discern what serves you in your relationships, career, and even your food choices.

Trauma, whether big or small, shapes us. We often carry these traumas for years, forming attachments to people or things to manage our unresolved pain. Understanding this helps us recognize when our stress personality appears and empowers us to choose how we respond. It's about reclaiming your power and deciding to live a life that's aligned with your true nature, free from the stories that have kept you stuck.

Shifting your eating habits in alignment with the circadian rhythm, practicing mindfulness, and managing the DMN can all contribute to inner harmony. Ego attachment to thoughts, beliefs, and desires can lead to imbalance, but a healthy ego fosters resilience and a sense of self free from attachments. As you release these attachments, your true, vibrant self emerges.

The three brain model—encompassing the CNS, ENS, and the microbiome—is an essential framework for achieving harmony. These three "brains" work together, influencing how you think, feel, and transform. When they align, your entire system functions optimally.

If you seek a more vibrant, energetic existence with optimal health, fulfilling relationships, and a purposeful life, then join me on this path. Together, we can heal, grow, and create a world where true health of mind, body, and spirit emerges. The journey is yours to take. Will you choose the well-worn path, or will you embark on the one less traveled? You hold the power to decide. I urge you not to simply close this book and return to a programmed life. The comfort zone will only prevent you from fully living an abundant, fulfilling life.

Remember this beautiful quote by the Sufi poet Rumi: "Yesterday I was clever, so I wanted to change the world. Today I am wise, so I am changing myself."

Thank you for being a part of this journey. It's for you that I share this work, and I feel blessed to pass on this wisdom.

Yours truly,
Trupti Gokani

Stay connected and stay in touch for upcoming events, lectures, workshops and more!

www.truptigokanimd.com

Facebook: www.facebook.com/TruptiGokaniMD

Instagram: www.instagram.com/drgokani/

LinkedIn: www.linkedin.com/in/trupti-gokani-md-17533a8/

Glossary

agni	Digestive fire
ahamkara	Ego, sense of identity
ajna chakra	The third eye
ama	An impaired bodily system that leads to toxicity
amygdala	Emotional processing, fear response center
anahata chakra	The heart chakra
anandamaya kosha	Bliss layer or kosha of your subtle body
annamaya kosha	Physical body layer or kosha of your subtle body
anterior cingulate cortex (ACC)	Emotional regulation center
asanas	Yoga poses
ashtanga yoga	Intense yoga

atma vichara	Soul analysis
autonomic nervous system (ANS)	Regulates involuntary functions
ayur	Life
Ayurveda	The ancient holistic science of self-healing
basal ganglia	Movement control, habit formation hub
bhajans	Prayer
bhakti yoga	Yogic path of devotion
bhava	Tenderness and love
bhujangasana	Cobra pose
Broca's region	The area of the temporal lobe associated with speech
buddhi	The intellect
chakra	Wheel representing life force energy
chitta	Cosmic intelligence
citta vrtti	Fluctuations of the mind
default mode network (DMN)	The part of the brain that is active when a person is at rest or mind-wandering
dharma	Living to your full potential
dhatus	Body tissues
dinacharya	Routines based on natural cycles
dosa	Indian crepes
dosha	Ayurvedic body type

enteric nervous system (ENS)	The nervous system in the gut
epigenetics	The impact of behavior, mindset, and environment on genes
guna	quality or tendency that is present in all living things
Ha	Sun
hatha yoga	Balanced yoga
hypothalamic-pituitary-adrenal axis	The neuroendocrine link between parts of the brain that respond to stress
hypothalamic-pituitary-adrenal maladaptation syndrome	Loss of internal hormone production rhythm due to remaining stuck in protective mode for too long
hypothalamus	Divine internal mother
ida	Nadis (channels of energy) on the right side of the body
jivatman	Soul's purpose
jnana yoga	The yogic path of higher wisdom
kapha	One of the three mind-body types (dosha) in Ayurveda
karma yoga	Yogic path of service
kensho	Japanese word for "seeing one's true nature"
kosha	Yogic term for sheaths or the layers of your being

kundalini	Feminine energy coiled like a snake at the base of the spine
kundalini yoga	Transformational yoga
lipopolysaccharide (LPS)	Cellular wall component of certain bacteria
malas	Wastes
manas	Mind
manipura chakra	The solar plexus chakra
manomaya kosha	Mind layer or kosha of your subtle body
maya	Illusions
medial prefrontal cortex (mPFC)	Controls the activity of the amygdala
muladhara chakra	The root chakra
nadi shodhana	Reverse nostril breathing
nadis	Meridians or channels of energy connecting chakras and running through bodily connective tissue
neuroception	The process of connecting to your nervous system
neurolinguistic programming (NLP)	Interdisciplinary field that studies how human brains process, understand, and produce language
neurological part	Different areas in the brain involved with memories, feelings, and reactions that may not be consciously remembered but serve as trauma triggers

parasympathetic nervous system (ParaNS)	Conserves resources
peripheral nervous system (PNS)	Nerves outside the brain and spinal cord
pingala	Nadis (channels of energy) on the right side of the body
pitta	One of the three mind-body types (dosha) in Ayurveda
pragyaparadh	Mistake of the intellect
prakruti	Birth nature or balanced birth energy state
prana	Life force energy, breath
pranamaya kosha	Breath layer or kosha of your subtle body
raja yoga	Yogic path of meditation
rajas	Infers a passionate or driven personality
reticular activating system (RAS)	Arousal regulation network in the brainstem
sahasrara chakra	The crown chakra
sat	Personal truth
satori	Japanese term for a sudden and profound experience of enlightenment or awakening that results in growth without pain
sattva	Infers a harmonious and calm personality
shakti	Divine feminine energy and power
sheaths	The kosha or layers comprising the subtle body

somatic nervous system	Regulates voluntary muscle function
subtle body	Thoughts, emotions, wisdom, and life force energy, linked to breath
sushumna	The main central nadis, also the center of the wheel of life
svadhisthana chakra	The sacral chakra
swathsa	Health
sympathetic nervous system (SNS)	Mobilizes resources
tamas	Infers a lazy or ignorant personality
Tha	Moon
trataka	Candle gazing
tridosha	The three biological energy sources governing bodily functions (vata, pitta, kapha)
vata	One of the three mind-body types (dosha) in Ayurveda
veda	Wisdom
vijnanamaya kosha	Intellect layer or kosha of your subtle body
vikruti	An unbalanced state that occurs when you make choices that push yourself out of alignment
vinyasa yoga	Flowing yoga
vishudda chakra	The throat chakra
yama	Control
yuj	To unify

Abbreviations

ACC	anterior cingulate cortex
ACTH	adrenocorticotropic hormone
AIM	Attention, intention, and meaning
aMPFC	anterior medial prefrontal cortex
ANS	autonomic nervous system
BDNF	brain-derived neurotrophic factor
CGRP	calcitonin gene-related peptide
CNS	central nervous system
DMN	default mode network
ENS	enteric nervous system
HPA	hypothalamic-pituitary-adrenal
LPS	lipopolysaccharide
MMC	migratory motor complex
MOW	model of the world
mPFC	medial prefrontal cortex
NLP	neurolinguistic programming
PCC	posterior cingulate cortex

PFC	prefrontal cortex
ParaNS	parasympathetic nervous system
PNS	peripheral nervous system
RAS	reticular activating system
SNS	sympathetic nervous system
SCM	subconscious mind
TPO	thyroid peroxidase
WHO	World Health Organization

Endnotes

Introduction

1   Office of the Actuary, "National Health Spending in 2020 Increases Due to Impact of COVID-19 Pandemic," CMS Press Release, December 15, 2021, https://www.cms.gov/newsroom/press-releases/national-health-spending-2020-increases-due-impact-covid-19-pandemic.

2   Micah Hartman, "Spending in 2018: Growth Driven by Accelerations in Medicare and Private Insurance Spending," *Health Affairs* 39, no. 1 (January 2020): 8–17, https://www.healthaffairs.org/doi/full/10.1377/hlthaff.2019.01451.

3   Charles H. Jones, Mikael Dolsten, "Healthcare on the Brink: Navigating the Challenges of an Aging Society in the United States," *Nature*, April 6, 2024, https://doi.org/10.1038/s41514-024-00148-2.

4   Matthew Griffin, "U.S. Healthcare Spending on Pace to Top $7 Trillion by 2031," *Los Angeles Times*, June 14, 2023, https://www.latimes.com/business/story/2023-06-14/u-s-healthcare-spending-on-pace-to-top-7-trillion-by-2031.

5   "Life Expectancy in the U.S. Dropped for the Second Year in a Row in 2021," CDC, National Center for Health Statistics, August 31, 2022, https://www.cdc.gov/nchs/pressroom/nchs_press_releases/2022/20220831.htm.

6   Trupti Gokani, MD, *The Mysterious Mind: How to Use Ancient Wisdom and Modern Science to Heal Your Headaches and Reclaim Your Health* (Silver Tree Communications, 2015).

Chapter 1

1   "WHO Remains Firmly Committed to the Principles Set Out in the Preamble to the Constitution," World Health Organization, accessed February 1, 2024, https://www.who.int/about/governance/constitution.

2   Antonio Damasio, *Descartes' Error: Emotion, Reason, and the Human Brain* (Grosset Putnam, 1994).

3   Annelise Madison, Janice K Kiecolt-Glaser, "Stress, Depression, Diet, and the Gut Microbiota: Human–Bacteria Interactions at the Core of Psychoneuroimmunology and Nutrition," *Current Opinion in Behavioral Sciences* 28 (August 2019): 105–110. https://www.ncbi.nlm.nih.gov/pmc/articles/PMC7213601/.

4   W. J. Strawbridge, et al, "Frequent Attendance at Religious Services and Mortality over 28 years," *American Journal of Public Health* 87, no. 6 (1997): 957–61.

5   H. G. Koenig, et al., "Attendance at Religious Services, Interleukin 6, and other Biological Parameters of Immune Function in Older Adults," *International Journal of Psychiatry in Medicine* 27 (1997): 233–50.

6   Tom Beckman, "Citations for 60-90% of All Doctor's Office Visits Are for Stress-Related Ailments and Complaints," LinkedIn, April 6, 2016, https://www.linkedin.com/pulse/citations-90-all-doctors-office-visits-stress-related-tom-beckman.

Chapter 2

1   "Stress Personality Quiz," Trupti Gokani, MD, www.truptigokanimd.com/stressrxbonus.

2   FactoryJoe, "Maslow's Hierarchy of Needs," Creative Commons, June 29, 2009, https://commons.wikimedia.org/wiki/File:Maslow%27s_Hierarchy_of_Needs.svg.

3   Mariam Arain, et al., "Maturation of the Adolescent Brain," *Neuropsychiatric Disease and Treatment* 9 (2013): 449–61. https://www.ncbi.nlm.nih.gov/pmc/articles/PMC3621648.

4   Emeran Mayer, "Gut Feelings: The Emerging Biology of Gut-Brain Communication," *Nature Reviews Neuroscience* 12 (2011): 453-66. https://www.nature.com/articles/nrn3071.

5   Michael D. Gershon, *The Second Brain: A Groundbreaking New Understanding of Nervous Disorders of the Stomach and Intestine* (Harper Perennial, 1999).

Chapter 3

1   "Energy," *Merriam-Webster Dictionary*, accessed December 22, 2024, https://www.merriam-webster.com/dictionary/energy.

2   "Energy," *Merriam-Webster*.

3   Bruce Lipton, *The Biology of Belief: Unleashing the Power of Consciousness, Matter, & Miracles* (Hay House, 2008).

4   Gabor Maté, *When the Body Says No: The Cost of Hidden Stress* (Vintage Canada, 2004).

5   Louise Hay, *You Can Heal Your Life* (Hay House, 1984).

6   Wayne W. Dyer, *Change Your Thoughts, Change Your Life: Living the Wisdom of the Tao* (Hay House, 2009).

7   Bruce Lipton, "Your Life Is a Printout of Your Subconscious Mind," Facebook, September 23, 2021, https://www.facebook.com/BruceHLiptonPhD/posts/95-percent-of-your-life-is-coming-from-a-subconscious-program-your-life-is-a-pri/4960784917269328/.

8   Max-Planck-Gesellschaft, "Decision-Making May Be Surprisingly Unconscious Activity," ScienceDaily, April 15, 2008, https://www.sciencedaily.com/releases/2008/04/080414145705.htm.

Chapter 4

1   Mihaly Csikszentmihalyi, *Flow: The Psychology of Optimal Experience* (Harper Perennial Modern Classics, 2008), 23–29.

Chapter 5

1   Michael T. Kinsella, "Impact of Mental Stress, Depression & Anxiety on Fetal Neurobehavioral Development," *Clinical Obstetrics and Gynecology* 52, no. 3 (September 2009): 425–40. https://journals.lww.com/clinicalobgyn/Abstract/2009/09000/Impact_of_Maternal_Stress,_Depression_and_Anxiety.16.aspx&.

2   N. M. Talge, et al., "Antenatal Maternal Stress and Long-Term Effects on Child Neurodevelopment: How and Why?," *Journal of Child Psychology and Psychiatry* 48, no 3-4 (2007): 245–61.

Chapter 6

1   C. Benet, "The Epidemiology of Traumatic Event Exposure Worldwide: Results from the World Mental Health Survey Consortium," *Psychological Medicine* 46, no. 2 (January 2016): 327–43.

2   Elisabet Sanchez-Rodriguez, "The Role of Self-Presentation in Pediatric Pain," *International Journal of Environmental Research and Public Health* 18, no. 2 (January 2021): 591. https://www.ncbi.nlm.nih.gov/pmc/articles/PMC7828281/.

3   Gabor Maté, *When the Body Says No: Exploring the Stress-Disease Connection* (John Wiley and Sons, 2011).

4   A. Hart, M. A. Kamm, "Mechanisms of Initiation and Perpetuation of Gut Inflammation by Stress," *Alimentary Pharmacology and Therapeutics* 16, no. 12 (December 2002): 2017–28. https://onlinelibrary.wiley.com/doi/abs/10.1046/j.1365-2036.2002.01359.x.

5   Lydia Saad, "Eight in 10 Americans Afflicted by Stress," Gallup News, December 20, 2017, https://news.gallup.com/poll/224336/eight-americans-afflicted-stress.aspx.

6   H. Hoel, et al., "The Cost of Violence/Stress at Work and the Benefits of a Violence/Stress-Free Working Environment," International Labour Organisation, January 1, 2001, https://www.ilo.org/publications/cost-violencestress-work-and-ben-efits-violencestress-free-working.

7   Juliet Hassard and Kevin Teoh, "The Cost of Work-Related Stress: A Systematic Review," *Journal of Occupational Health Psychology* 23, no. 1 (March 2017): 1–17. https://www.researchgate.net/publication/313480340_The_cost_of_work-related_stress_a_systematic_review.

8   Enes Sarigedik, et al., "Intergenerational Transmission of Psychological Trauma: A Structural Neuroimaging Study," *Psychiatry Research: Neuroimaging* 326 (October 2022). https://www.sciencedirect.com/science/article/abs/pii/S0925492722000993.

Chapter 7

1   Karl Albrecht, *Stress and the Manager* (Touchstone, 1986).

2   Gabriel A. Orenstein and Lindsay Lewis, "Erikson's Stages of Psychosocial Development," National Library of Medicine, updated November 7, 2022, https://www.ncbi.nlm.nih.gov/books/NBK556096/.

3   Stephen W. Porges, *The Pocket Guide to the Polyvagal Theory* (W. W. Norton & Company, 2017).

Chapter 8

1   Michael Bernard Beckwith, "The 4 Stages of Spiritual Awakening," uploaded by MindValley, June 21, 2018, YouTube, 4:08, https://www.youtube.com/watch?v=vg-D2DMFbhk.

2   Viktor E. Frankl discusses this concept in *Man's Search for Meaning* (Beacon Press, 2006), 75–84.

3   Harold G. Koenig, "Religion and Medicine 1: Historical Background and Reasons for Separation," *International Journal of Psychiatry in Medicine* 30, no. 4 (2000): 385–98.

4   R. A. Hummer, et al., "Religious Involvement and US Adult Mortality," *Demography* 36 (1999): 273–85.

5   Olga Herren, et al., "Influence of Spirituality on Depression-Induced Inflammation and Executive Functioning in a Community Sample of African Americans," *Ethnicity and Disease* 29, no. 2 (Spring 2019): 267–27. https://www.ncbi.nlm.nih.gov/pmc/articles/PMC6478044/.

6   Alia J Crum, et al., "Mind Over Milkshakes: Mindsets, Not Just Nutrients, Determine Ghrelin Response," *Health Psychology* 30, no. 4 (July 2011): 424–29. https://pubmed.ncbi.nlm.nih.gov/21574706/.

7   Sarah Lohman, *Eight Flavors: The Untold Story of American Cuisine* (Simon & Schuster, 2017).

8   Isabel E. Young, et al., "Distribution of Energy Intake Across the Day and Weight Loss: A Systematic Review and Meta-Analysis," *Obesity Reviews* 24,no. 3 (March 2023): e13537. https://onlinelibrary.wiley.com/doi/10.1111/obr.13537; Chenjuan Gu, et al., "Metabolic Effects of Late Dinner in Healthy Volunteers-A Randomized Crossover Clinical Trial," *Journal of Clinical Endocrinology & Metabolism* 105, no. 8 (August 2020): 2789–802.

9   Press Release, Nobel Foundation, October 2, 2017, https://www.nobelprize.org/prizes/medicine/2017/press-release/.

10   Xuhui Luo, "Seasonal Change in Microbial Diversity and Its Relationship with Soil Chemical Properties in an Orchard," *PLOS One* 14, no. 12 (2019): e0215556. https://www.ncbi.nlm.nih.gov/pmc/articles/PMC6938340/; Samuel A. Smits, et al., "Seasonal Cycling in the Gut Microbiome of the Hadza Hunter-Gatherers of Tanzania," *Science* 357, no. 6353 (August 2017): 802–6.

Chapter 9

1   Marcus E Raichle and Abraham Z Snyder, "A Default Mode of Brain Function: A Brief History of an Evolving Idea," *Neuroimage* 37, no. 4 (2007): 1083–90. https://pubmed.ncbi.nlm.nih.gov/17719799/.

2   R. L. Buckner, et al., "The Brain's Default Network: Anatomy, Function, and Relevance to Disease," *Annals of the New York Academy of Sciences* 1124, no. 1 (2008): 1–38.

3   Tina Chou, et al., "The Default Mode Network and Rumination in Individuals at Risk for Depression," *Social Cognitive and Affective Neuroscience* 18, no. 1 (2023): nsad032. https://academic.oup.com/scan/article/18/1/nsad032/7188150.

4   Randy L. Buckner, "The Serendipitous Discovery of the Brain's Default Network," *Neuroimage* 62, no. 2 (2012): 1137–45. 10.1016/j.neuroimage.2011.10.035.

5   Robert S. Weiss, *Loneliness: The Experience of Emotional and Social Isolation* (The MIT Press, 1975).

6   National Academies of Sciences, Engineering, and Medicine, *Social Isolation and Loneliness in Older Adults* (The National Academies Press, 2020), https://doi.org/10.17226/25663.

7   Daniel S. Barron and Stephanie Yarnell, "Default Mode Network: The Basics for Psychiatrists," *Fundamentals of Neuroscience in Psychiatry*, National Neuroscience Curriculum Initiative, accessed December 23, 2024, https://www.nncionline.org/wp-content/uploads/2015/12/DMN_p4.pdf.

Chapter 10

1   "About Central Council of Indian Medicine," Central Council of Indian Medicine, accessed May 24, 2024, https://www.ccimindia.org.in/introduction/.

2   "Stress Personality Quiz," Trupti Gokani, MD, www.truptigokanimd.com/stress-rxbonus.

3   Although these words are frequently attributed to Ralph Waldo Emerson, they're believed to be a paraphrase or adaptation of ideas that resonate with Emerson's philosophy, rather than a direct quote from his works. They may instead be the words of Bessie A. Stanley from an essay written circa 1905, see Quote Investigator, June 6, 2012, https://quoteinvestigator.com/2012/06/26/define-success/.

Chapter 11

1   Robert W. Levenson, "Blood, Sweat, and Fears: The Autonomic Architecture of Emotion," in "Emotions Inside Out: 130 Years after Darwin's The Expression of the Emotions in Man and Animals. Part IV. Physiology," *Annals of the New York Academy of Sciences* 1000, no. 1 (2003): 348–66. https://doi.org/10.1196/annals.1280.016.

2   "German New Medicine Therapy," Med Rehab Group, accessed December 23, 2024, https://medrehabgroup.com/physiotherapy-center-treatments/german-new-medicine-therapy/.

3   Bernie Siegel, *Love, Medicine & Miracles: Lessons Learned about Self-Healing from a Surgeon's Experience with Exceptional Patients* (William Morrow, 1998), 79–84.

4   Sir David Hawkins, *Power vs. Force* (Hay House, 2002).

5   Michael D. Gershon, *The Second Brain: A Groundbreaking New Understanding of Nervous Disorders of the Stomach and Intestine* (Harper Perennial, 1999).

6   Annelise Madison and Janice K Kiecolt-Glaser, "Stress, Depression, Diet, and the Gut Microbiota: Human-Bacteria Interactions at the Core of Psychoneuroimmunology and Nutrition," *Current Opinion in Behavioral Sciences* 28 (2019): 105–110. https://doi.org/10.1016/j.cobeha.2019.01.011.

7   Femke Lutgendorff, et al., "The Role of Microbiota and Probiotics in Stress-Induced Gastrointestinal Damage," *Current Molecular Medicine* 8 (2008): 282–98. https://doi.org/10.2174/156652408784533779.

8   Paul Ian Cross, "Do Gut Bacteria Play a Role in Depression?," Medical News Today, December 12, 2022, https://www.medicalnewstoday.com/articles/do-gut-bacteria-play-a-role-in-depression.

9   A. Allen, et al., "Bifidobacterium longum 1714 as a Translational Psychobiotic: Modulation of Stress, Electrophysiology and Neurocognition in Healthy Volunteers," *Translational Psychiatry* 6 (2016): e939. https://doi.org/10.1038/tp.2016.191.

10   P. Bercik, et al., "The Intestinal Microbiota Affect Central Levels of Brain-Derived Neurotropic Factor and Behavior in Mice," *Gastroenterology* 141, no. 2 (August 2011): 599–609. https://doi.org/10.1053/j.gastro.2011.04.052.

11   R. Savica, et al., "When Does Parkinson Disease Start?" *Archives of Neurology* 67, no. 7 (2010): 798–801. https://doi.org/10.1001/archneurol.2010.135; R. Savica, et al., "Medical Records Documentation of Constipation Preceding Parkinson's Disease: A Case-Control Study," *Neurology* 73 (2009):1752–1758. https://doi.org/10.1212/WNL.0b013e3181c34af5.

12   Jacob Horsager, et al., "Brain-First Versus Body-First Parkinson's Disease: A Multimodal Imaging Case-Control Study," *Brain* 143, no. 10 (October 2020): 3077–88. https://doi.org/10.1093/brain/awaa238.

13   Gabby Bernstein, *The Universe Has Your Back: Transform Fear to Faith* (Hay House, 2016).

14   Katrina Debnam, et al., "The Role of Stress and Spirituality in Adolescent Substance Use," *Substance Use & Misuse* 51, no. 6 (2016): 733–41. https://doi.org/10.3109 /10826084.2016.1155224.

15   Agnieszka Bożek, et al., "The Relationship Between Spirituality, Health-Related Behavior, and Psychological Well-Being," *Frontiers in Psychology* 11 (August 2020). https://doi.org/10.3389/fpsyg.2020.01997; Kwi Yun, et al., "Stress and Impact of Spirituality as a Mediator of Coping Methods among Social Work College Students," *Journal of Human Behavior in the Social Environment* 29, no. 1 (2019): 125–36. https://doi.org/10.1080/10911359.2018.1491918.

16   H. G. Koenig, et al., "Attendance at Religious Services, Interleukin 6, and Other Biological Parameters of Immune Function in Older Adults," *International Journal of Psychiatry in Medicine* 27 (1997): 233–50; W. J. Strawbridge, et al, "Frequent Attendance at Religious Services and Mortality over 28 years," *American Journal of Public Health* 87, no. 6 (1997): 957–61.

Chapter 12

1   Vasant Lad, *Ayurveda: The Science of Self-Healing* (Lotus Press, 1984), 40.

2   Nayyirah Waheed, *Salt* (CreateSpace Independent Publishing Platform, 2013).

3   Daniel Goleman, *Emotional Intelligence: Why It Can Matter More Than IQ*, 10th anniversary ed. (Bantam, 2005).

4   Masoumeh Shohani, et al., "The Effect of Yoga on Stress, Anxiety, and Depression in Women," *International Journal of Preventive Medicine* 9, no. 1 (2018): 21. https://doi.org/10.4103/ijpvm.IJPVM_242_16.

5   Fu-Jung Huang, et al., "Effects of Hatha Yoga on Stress in Middle-Aged Women," *Journal of Nursing Research* 21, no. 1 (March 2013): 59–66. https://doi.org/10.1097/ jnr.0b013e3182829d6d.

6   Sarah Murphy, "Is There Scientific Evidence for the Chakras?," Association for Comprehensive Energy Psychology Blog, September 1, 2022, https://www.energypsych.org/blog/is-there-scientific-evidence-for-the-chakras.

7   Tias Little, *Yoga of the Subtle Body: A Guide to the Physical and Energetic Anatomy of Yoga* (Shambala, 2016), 109.

8   Dian Land, "Study Shows Compassion Meditation Changes the Brain," University of Wisconsin-Madison News, March 25, 2008, https://news.wisc.edu/study-shows-compassion-meditation-changes-the-brain/.

Chapter 13

1   Diane Feskanich, et al., "Milk Consumption During Teenage Years and Risk of Hip Fractures in Older Adults," *JAMA Pediatrics* 168, no. 1 (2014): 54–60. https://doi.org/10.1001/jamapediatrics.2013.3821.

2   Stephen R. Covey, *The 7 Habits of Highly Effective People* (Simon and Schuster, 1990).

3   For more on this, see *The Mysterious Mind*, Chapter 4, "Understanding Your Body's Body Chemistry."

4   Nuraly S. Akimbekov, et al., "Vitamin D and the Host-Gut Microbiome: A Brief Overview," *Acta Histochemica et Cytochemica* 53, no. 3 (2020): 33–42. https://doi.org/10.1267/ahc.20011.

5   P. Singh, et al., "The Potential Role of Vitamin D Supplementation as a Gut Microbiota Modifier in Healthy Individuals," *Scientific Reports* 10 (2020). https://doi.org/10.1038/s41598-020-77806-4.

6   Ş. Akpınar and M. G. Karadağ, "Is Vitamin D Important in Anxiety or Depression? What Is the Truth?," *Current Nutrition Reports* 11 (2022): 675–81. https://doi.org/10.1007/s13668-022-00441-0.

7   Michael Camilleri, "Leaky Gut: Mechanisms, Measurement and Clinical Implications in Humans," *Gut* 68 (2019):1516-1526. https://gut.bmj.com/content/68/8/1516.share.

8   Y. Li Y, et al., "Gut Microbiota Changes and Their Relationship with Inflammation in Patients with Acute and Chronic Insomnia," *Nature and Science of Sleep* 12 (2020): 895–905. https://doi.org/10.2147/NSS.S271927; F. Benhadou, et al., "Psoriasis and Microbiota: A Systematic Review," *Diseases* 6, no. 2 (2018):47. https://doi.org/10.3390/diseases6020047; Melanie Schirmer, "Linking the Human Gut Microbiome to Inflammatory Cytokine Production Capacity," *Cell* 167, no. 4 (November 2016): 1125-1136. https://doi.org/10.1016/j.cell.2016.10.020.

9   G.Y. Liu and D. M. Sabatini, "mTOR at the Nexus of Nutrition, Growth, Ageing and Disease," *Nature Reviews Molecular Cell Biology* 21 (2020): 183–203. https://doi.org/10.1038/s41580-019-0199-y.

10   A. Allen, et al., "Bifidobacterium longum 1714 as a Translational Psychobiotic: Modulation of Stress, Electrophysiology and Neurocognition in Healthy Volunteers," *Translational Psychiatry* 6 (2016): e939. https://doi.org/10.1038/tp.2016.191.

11   E. Zaura, et al., "Same Exposure But Two Radically Different Responses to Antibiotics: Resilience of the Salivary Microbiome Versus Long-Term Microbial Shifts in Feces," *mBio* 6, no. 6 (2015). https://doi.org/10.1128/mBio.01693-15.

12   "FDA Drug Safety Communication: Prescription Acetaminophen Products to be Limited to 325 mg Per Dosage Unit; Boxed Warning Will Highlight Potential for Severe Liver Failure," US Food & Drug Administration, January 13, 2011, https://www.fda.gov/drugs/drug-safety-and-availability/fda-drug-safety-communication-prescription-acetaminophen-products-be-limited-325-mg-dosage-unit.

13   "FDA Drug Safety Communication: Low magnesium levels can be associated with long-term use of Proton Pump Inhibitor drugs (PPIs)," US Food & Drug Administration, March 2, 2011, https://www.fda.gov/drugs/drug-safety-and-availability/fda-drug-safety-communication-low-magnesium-levels-can-be-associated-long-term-use-proton-pump.

14   Zawn Villines, "What to Know about H2 Blockers," Medical News Today, February 10, 2023, https://www.medicalnewstoday.com/articles/h2-blockers#when-to-avoid.

15   Z. Al-Aly, et al., "Proton Pump Inhibitors and the Kidney: Implications of Current Evidence for Clinical Practice and When and How to Deprescribe," *American Journal of Kidney Diseases* 75, no. 4 (April 2020): 497–507. https://doi.org/10.1053/j.ajkd.2019.07.012.

16   A. M. Valdes, et al., "Role of the Gut Microbiota in Nutrition and Health," *BMJ* (2018): 361:k2179. https://doi.org/10.1136/bmj.k2179; Jiyoung Kim, et al., "Naturally Occurring Phytochemicals for the Prevention of Alzheimer's Disease," *Journal of Neurochemistry* 112, no. 6 (February 2010): 1415–1430. https://doi.org/10.1111/j.1471-4159.2009.06562.x.

9 781964 686363